Essential Prescribing

Other titles from Scion

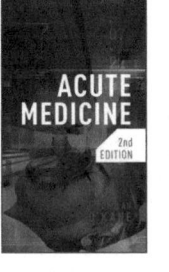 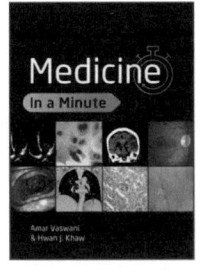 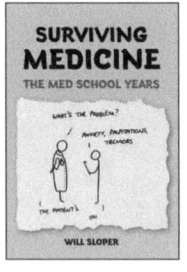 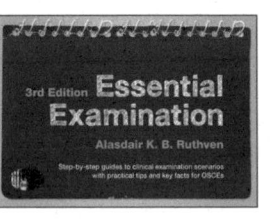 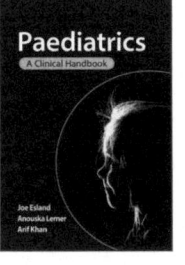 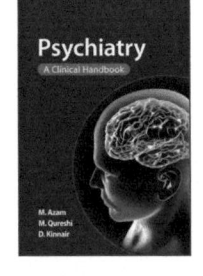 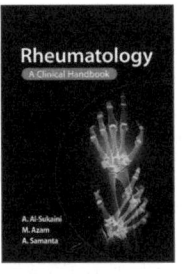

Scion

Essential Prescribing

**A guide to the most
common drugs in medicine**

Razan Nour

MB BCh, BAO
Foundation Year 2 Doctor, Northern Deanery

First published 2018

ISBN 9781911510000

A CIP catalogue record for this book is available from the British Library.

Scion Publishing Limited

The Old Hayloft, Vantage Business Park, Bloxham Road, Banbury, Oxfordshire OX16 9UX

www.scionpublishing.com

Important Note from the Publisher

The information contained within this book was obtained by Scion Publishing Limited from sources believed by us to be reliable. However, while every effort has been made to ensure its accuracy, no responsibility for loss or injury whatsoever occasioned to any person acting or refraining from action as a result of information contained herein can be accepted by the author or publishers.

Readers should remember that medicine is a constantly evolving science and while the author and publishers have ensured that all dosages, applications and practices are based on current indications, there may be specific practices which differ between communities. You should always follow the guidelines laid down by the manufacturers of specific products and the relevant authorities in the country in which you are practising.

Although every effort has been made to ensure that all owners of copyright material have been acknowledged in this publication, we would be pleased to acknowledge in subsequent reprints or editions any omissions brought to our attention.

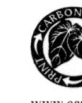 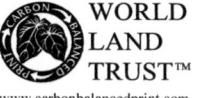

www.carbonbalancedprint.com
CBP2250

Typeset by Medlar Publishing Services Pvt Ltd, India

Printed in the UK

Last digit is the print number: 10 9 8

CONTENTS

DETAILED CONTENTS LIST

PREFACE

I started thinking about developing a book on prescribing while still a final year medical student, and I started writing shortly after my finals. I was inspired by *Essential Examination* by Alasdair Ruthven (also from Scion Publishing), which is a very popular and widely used systems-based guide to clinical examination. The concise short-note format of *Essential Examination* was particularly useful for exam revision and I thought that it might be possible to emulate its style and format and apply this to pharmacology and safe prescribing. Hopefully, my approach will make the experience of studying these subjects more tolerable for those who find them dry and boring. But you must study them! Safe prescribing is highly topical and, in the UK, the GMC has introduced the Prescribing Safety Assessment as a compulsory examination that final year medical students must pass in order to practise as junior doctors.

Essential Prescribing comprises two sections: 'Prescribing by system' and 'Prescribing by situation'. It contains dedicated entries to the most frequently prescribed medications in medicine, including emergency drugs, and it addresses prescribing in individuals who are elderly, pregnant or suffering from renal impairment. It provides easy access to the need-to-know facts about each drug, using a consistent structure throughout:

- examples of each type of drug
- mode of action
- indications and contraindications
- monitoring
- side-effects
- patient counselling.

In addition, I have kept descriptions short, used mnemonics where possible to help memorise important information, and provided space for your own notes. Sign-posting to relevant guidelines is also provided.

I am confident that this book will help students revising for the PSA exam by providing a solid foundation of knowledge about pharmacology and prescribing. If you have any views about this book that you would like to share or any suggestions on how to improve it for the future, feel free to contact me on essentialprescribing2017@gmail.com.

I hope that you find this book as useful as I have intended!

Razan Nour
January 2018

ACKNOWLEDGMENTS

I am very grateful to Sadia Qayyum (pharmacist and lecturer in pharmacy practice at the University of Manchester) for her thorough review of the manuscript, and to Laura Hartley, current medical student and qualified pharmacist, for providing further input on the manuscript (it was invaluable to gain input from someone with a medical student perspective but with knowledge and practical experience in pharmacy). Furthermore, I appreciate the feedback and suggestions provided by Scion Publishing's student review panel which helped to shape this book.

I would like to take the opportunity to thank my family and my friends for their undying support and encouragement whilst writing this book and during my journey from medical school to working as a junior doctor.

Finally, I would like to thank the staff at Scion Publishing for the care and attention this work received during the publication process – it was second to none.

ABBREVIATIONS

A&E	Accident and Emergency		CXR	chest X-ray
ABG	arterial blood gas		DCT	distal convoluted tubule
ACE	angiotensin-converting enzyme		DEXA	dual energy X-ray absorptiometry
ACEi	ACE inhibitors		DHF	dihydrofolic acid
AChEi	acetylcholinesterase inhibitors		DOAC	direct oral anticoagulant
ACS	acute coronary syndrome		DVLA	Driver and Vehicle Licensing Agency
ADH	antidiuretic hormone		DVT	deep vein thrombosis
ADP	adenosine diphosphate		ECF	extracellular fluid
ADR	adverse drug reaction		ECG	electrocardiogram
AF	atrial fibrillation		ECT	electroconvulsive therapy
AKI	acute kidney injury		eGFR	estimated GFR
ALT	alanine transaminase		EPSE	extrapyramidal side-effects
AMP	adenosine monophosphate		FBC	full blood count
ARB	angiotensin receptor blocker/antagonist		FMF	familial Mediterranean fever
AV	arteriovenous		FSH	follicle-stimulating hormone
BiPAP	bilevel positive airway pressure		GABA	gamma-aminobutyric acid
BMI	body mass index		GCS	Glasgow Coma Score
BP	blood pressure		GFR	glomerular filtration rate
BPH	benign prostatic hypertrophy		GI	gastrointestinal
cAMP	cyclic AMP		GMP	guanosine monophosphate
CCB	calcium channel blocker		GORD	gastro-oesophageal reflux disease
cGMP	cyclic GMP		GP	General Practitioner
CHM	Commission on Human Medicines		GTN	glyceryl trinitrate
CI	contraindication		HDL	high-density lipoprotein
CK	creatine kinase		HF	heart failure
CMV	cytomegalovirus		HIT	heparin-induced thrombocytopenia
CNS	central nervous system		HMG CoA	hydroxymethylglutaryl coenzyme A
COCP	combined oral contraceptive pill		HONK	hyperglycaemic hyperosmolar non-ketotic coma
COPD	chronic obstructive pulmonary disease		HPA	hypothalamic–pituitary–adrenal
COX	cyclo-oxygenase		HR	heart rate
CPAP	continuous positive airway pressure		HTN	hypertension
CPR	cardiopulmonary resuscitation		IBD	inflammatory bowel disease
CrCl	creatinine clearance		ICF	intracellular fluid
CRP	C-reactive protein		IHD	ischaemic heart disease
CVA	cerebrovascular accident		IM	intramuscular
CVD	cardiovascular disease		INR	international normalized ratio

ISDN	isosorbide dinitrate
ISMN	isosorbide mononitrate
IV	intravenous
JVP	jugular venous pressure
LA	local anaesthetic
LABA	long-acting beta-2 adrenoceptor agonist
LAMA	long-acting muscarinic antagonist
LFTs	liver function tests
LH	luteinizing hormone
LV	left ventricle
MAOI	monoamine oxidase inhibitor
MHRA	Medicines and Healthcare products Regulatory Agency
MI	myocardial infarction
MMSE	Mini Mental State Examination
MOVU	minimum obligatory volume of urine
MRSA	methicillin-resistant *Staphylococcus aureus*
MSK	musculoskeletal
NAC	*N*-acetylcysteine
NAPQI	*N*-acetyl-*p*-benzoquinone imine
NEWS	National Early Warning Score
NG	nasogastric
NICE	National Institute for Health and Care Excellence
NMDA	*N*-methyl-D-aspartate
NO	nitric oxide
NOAC	novel oral anticoagulant
NSAID	non-steroidal anti-inflammatory drug
OAB	overactive bladder
PCA	patient-controlled analgesia
PCOS	polycystic ovarian syndrome
PCT	proximal convoluted tubule

PD	Parkinson's disease
PE	pulmonary embolism
PEFR	peak expiratory flow rate
PO	per os (by mouth)
POP	progestogen-only pill
PPI	proton pump inhibitor
PR	per rectum
PSA	prostate-specific antigen / Prescribing Safety Assessment
RAAS	renin–angiotensin–aldosterone system
RR	respiratory rate
SABA	short-acting beta-2 adrenoceptor agonist
SAMA	short-acting muscarinic antagonist
S/C	subcutaneous
SSRI	selective serotonin reuptake inhibitor
STI	sexually transmitted infection
SUDEP	sudden unexpected death in epilepsy
SVT	supraventricular tachycardia
TCA	tricyclic antidepressant
TEN	toxic epidermal necrolysis
TFTs	thyroid function tests
THF	tetrahydrofolic acid
TIA	transient ischaemic attack
TPN	total parenteral nutrition
U+Es	urea and electrolytes
UTI	urinary tract infection
VF	ventricular fibrillation
VT	ventricular tachycardia
VTE	venous thromboembolism
WCC	white cell count
WPW	Wolff–Parkinson–White syndrome

GENERAL PRESCRIBING RULES

Below is a list of 'rules' to encourage safe prescribing:

1. All prescriptions must include name of drug, route of delivery, dose and frequency. If prescribing an as-required medication, also include the dosing interval and the maximum dose in 24 hours. The prescriber must sign and date each prescription.
2. Use a current list of the patient's medications before prescribing and confirm with the patient or the patient's carer that the patient is taking each medication that is prescribed on admission. The patient's GP can be a good source of information if medication queries arise.
3. **ALWAYS** ask about and document known allergies and type of reaction. Note that this applies not only to drug allergies; other allergies, such as to food and to material (e.g. latex), are also relevant.
4. If the patient is taking insulin, ensure that the correct type of insulin pen that the patient normally uses is also prescribed. Using the wrong insulin pen can result in drug errors.
5. It is good practice to check the patient's blood glucose before prescribing an insulin dose. Seek senior help or contact the local diabetes team for advice if it is a challenge to obtain satisfactory glycaemic control in a specific patient.
6. **NEVER** abbreviate the word 'UNITS' in an insulin prescription.
7. **NEVER** abbreviate the word 'micrograms' to 'mcg'.
8. It is the prescriber's responsibility to ensure that there are no dangerous interactions that may cause harm between any new medication that the patient is being prescribed and the patient's regular medications.
9. **REVIEW** the need to continue medications, particularly PRN medications, as the patient might not have required some of their medications whilst in hospital.
10. **REVIEW** the patient's fluid status and their most recent blood results before prescribing IV fluids. In some cases, it might be necessary to stop IV fluid administration.
11. Potassium should **NEVER** be added to intravenous fluid bags containing potassium (e.g. Hartmann's solution) as this is dangerous (may result in hyperkalaemia).
12. Ensure that it is clear on the discharge medication script which medications the patient should continue after discharge and for how long. Please include this information in the discharge letter to the GP, if relevant, as it is the GP who will continue to manage the patient's chronic conditions in the community.
13. If the patient is being prescribed any new devices for administration of medications, e.g. inhalers for respiratory problems or auto-injector devices for anaphylaxis, the patient should receive teaching on correct use of the specific device they are being prescribed and the prescriber should be satisfied that the patient is able to use the device safely.
14. If a patient is being started on a new medication, the prescriber should **COUNSEL** the patient on the drug's side-effects and the patient must be informed of dangerous or life-threatening adverse effects. The prescriber should document the information that they have informed the patient. Failure to counsel patients sufficiently and to provide documentation of this may constitute clinical negligence and compromise a doctor's medico-legal defence in the event of a serious incident.

NOTES ON UNITS

- Always spell out in full the word **MICROGRAMS** rather than abbreviate it to either 'μg' or 'mcg'. This is to avoid the possibility of misinterpreting 'mcg' as 'mg', and thereby giving the patient a much higher dose (by a factor of 1000).
- Always spell out in full the word **UNITS** when prescribing insulin. For patient safety reasons it is strongly discouraged to abbreviate international units to 'IU', as these letters could be misread as numbers if handwriting is poor.

Section I:
Prescribing by system

ACE inhibitors (ACEi)

Examples	• Captopril, enalapril, lisinopril, perindopril, ramipril	→ End in -pril
Mode of action	• Inhibit conversion of angiotensin 1 to angiotensin 2 by blocking angiotensin-converting enzyme (ACE)	→ Angiotensin 2 is a potent vasoconstrictor, hence blocking its production causes blood vessels to relax and dilate
Route of delivery	• PO	→ Combination drugs containing ACEi with CCBs or diuretics exist to make it easier for patients who take multiple medications to control their blood pressure
Indications	• Hypertension • Chronic heart failure • Ischaemic heart disease • Diabetic nephropathy (not in renal impairment)	→ 1st line in Caucasian people and those aged <55 (NICE 2011, CG127) → 1st line in chronic heart failure → One of the five drugs indicated post-MI (NICE 2013, CG172) → Slows progression of renovascular disease
Cautions and contraindications	• Renal artery stenosis or known renal impairment • Known hypersensitivity • Hyperkalaemia • Women who are pregnant (ACEi should be avoided throughout pregnancy) • Seek specialist advice before using in aortic stenosis, mitral stenosis and hypertrophic cardiomyopathy • Some ACEi should be avoided in breastfeeding but others are deemed safe for use	→ ACEi reduce glomerular filtration → Teratogenic: damages fetal renal function and BP control → ACEi cause vasodilatation which can cause blood pressure reduction in these fixed cardiac outputs
Monitoring	• Check U+Es prior to starting treatment and 1–2 weeks after, and on increasing dose	→ To establish baseline renal function
Interactions	• Nephrotoxic: NSAIDs, lithium, metformin, diuretics • K⁺-sparing diuretics and K⁺ supplements • Other drugs affecting the renin–angiotensin–aldosterone system (RAAS)	→ Increased risk of AKI → Increased risk of hyperkalaemia → Increased risk of hypotension, hyperkalaemia and renal impairment compared to the use of a single drug

Side-effects	• Common:
	  – Dry cough (because ACEi inhibit bradykinin metabolism and free bradykinins cause bronchoconstriction)
	  – 1st dose hypotension
	  – Hyperkalaemia
	• Less common:
	  – Angioedema (very rare but important for patients to be aware of)
		• Mnemonic **CAPTOPRIL (ACEi side-effects)**
		Cough
		Anaphylaxis (or **A**ngioedema)
		Palpitations
		Taste disturbance
		Orthostatic hypotension
		Potassium elevated
		Renal impairment
		Impotence
		Leucocytosis

Patient counselling	• **Dry cough:**	→	If the patient develops dry cough within the first months of starting ACEi they should report this to their GP and the drug should be switched to an ARB.
	• **1st dose hypotension:**	→	If the patient is at risk of 1st dose hypotension suggest that dose is taken at night.
	• **NSAIDs:**	→	Do not take non-steroidal anti-inflammatory medications (e.g. ibuprofen) when taking this drug.
	• **Surgery:**	→	ACEi are normally stopped on the day of surgery (unless told otherwise).
	• **Pregnancy:**	→	If the patient becomes pregnant, the ACEi must be stopped immediately (preferably within 2 working days of notification of pregnancy) and alternatives offered (NICE 2010, CG107).
	• **Angioedema/allergic reaction:**	→	If swelling of the face, eyes, lips or tongue develops or if breathing difficulties occur, stop drug and call an ambulance.

Angiotensin receptor antagonists (also known as angiotensin receptor blockers – ARBs)

Examples	• Candesartan, irbesartan, losartan, valsartan	→ End in -sartan
Mode of action	• Block action of angiotensin II on the AT_1 receptor	→ Angiotensin 2 is a potent vasoconstrictor, hence blocking its action allows blood vessels to relax and dilate
Routes of delivery	• PO	
Indications	Same as ACEi, 2nd line if ACEi not tolerated: • Hypertension • Chronic heart failure • Ischaemic heart disease and post-MI • Diabetic nephropathy	→ Does not cause dry cough (unlike ACEi) → Lower doses should be used in renal impairment
Cautions and contraindications	Same cautions and contraindications as ACEi, [p. 2 for more information], with the exception that some ARBs are contraindicated in severe hepatic impairment	• Mnemonic **PARK (ACEi and ARB cautions and CI)** **P**regnancy **A**llergy **R**enal artery stenosis **K**+ elevated (hyperkalaemia)
Interactions	• Same as ACEi [p. 2]	
Monitoring	• U+Es before and 1–2 weeks after starting treatment	→ To establish baseline renal function

Side-effects	• Common:
	  – 1st dose hypotension
	• Less common:
	  – Hyperkalaemia, renal impairment, angioedema	

Patient counselling	• ***No dry cough:*** explain that drug does not cause dry cough but may cause dizziness and hyperkalaemia. • ***NSAIDs:*** NSAIDs should not be used with this drug. • ***Pregnancy:*** if the patient becomes pregnant, the ARB must be stopped immediately (preferably within 2 working days of notification of pregnancy) and alternatives offered (NICE 2010, CG107).	→ ACEi prevent metabolism of bradykinins whereas ARBs do not influence bradykinin breakdown → Increased risk of renal impairment → Teratogenic: damages fetal renal function and BP control

Beta-adrenoceptor blocking drugs (beta blockers)

Examples	• Cardioselective: atenolol, bisoprolol, celiprolol, metoprolol, acebutolol	→ End in -lol; primarily target beta-adrenoceptors in the heart (cause fewer effects on organs outside heart)
	• Not cardioselective: nadolol, oxprenolol, propranolol, sotalol, timolol	→ End in -lol; target beta-adrenoceptors in the heart and other organs
Mode of action	• Inhibit stimulation of beta-adrenoceptors in the heart (if selective) and in vascular smooth muscle, bronchi and other organs e.g. liver and pancreas (if non-selective)	→ Beta blockade on the heart results in a reduction of heart rate and force of contraction
		→ Beta blockade outside the heart causes vasoconstriction and bronchoconstriction
Routes of delivery	• PO • IV (e.g. IV metoprolol in atrial fibrillation) • Topical (e.g. for treatment of glaucoma)	
Indications	• Hypertension • Chronic heart failure (not acute heart failure) • Ischaemic heart disease, especially post-MI prophylaxis and treatment of angina • Atrial fibrillation, atrial flutter and supraventricular tachycardia • Anxiety (propranolol) • Migraine • Thyrotoxicosis • Primary open angle glaucoma	→ Labetalol is used for hypertensive control in pregnancy, including gestational hypertension and pre-eclampsia → Beta blockers can cause a deterioration in acute HF → One of the five drugs indicated post-MI (NICE 2013, CG172)
Cautions and contraindications	• Asthma or COPD (risk of bronchospasm) – asthma is an absolute contraindication! • 2nd or 3rd degree heart block • Sick sinus syndrome • Uncontrolled heart failure • Bradycardia or hypotension • Hyperkalaemia • Metabolic acidosis • Severe peripheral arterial disease • **Use with caution in diabetic patients** and warn them that beta blockers may mask the signs of a hypoglycaemic attack (e.g. a diabetic patient might not experience signs of hypoglycaemia such as palpitations or tremor, due to beta blocker therapy)	→ If beta blocker use is required, a cardioselective type could be used under close supervision • Mnemonic **ABCDE (Beta blocker main contraindications and cautions)** **A**sthma **B**lock (heart block) **C**OPD **D**iabetes mellitus **E**lectrolytes (hyperkalaemia and metabolic acidosis)
Interactions	• Other anti-hypertensive drugs • Verapamil	→ Concurrent treatment may lead to hypotension → Complete heart block or significant blood pressure drop can occur – do not give IV verapamil within 8 hours of taking a beta blocker (Richards and Aronson, *Oxford Handbook of Practical Drug Therapy*, 2005, p. 144)

Beta-adrenoceptor blocking drugs (beta blockers) – *cont'd*

Monitoring	• Monitor the lung function of patients with obstructive airways disease who are taking beta blockers	

Side-effects	• Common:
	  – Fatigue
	  – Headache
	  – Dizziness
	  – Erectile dysfunction
	  – Sleep disturbances and nightmares
	  – Cold peripheries
	• Less common:
	  – May worsen Raynaud's disease
		→ Note that beta blockers vary in their degree of water or lipid solubility, which results in slightly different adverse effect profiles. Beta blockers that are more water soluble e.g. atenolol, nadolol and sotalol are less likely to cross the blood–brain barrier and cause less disturbance to sleep (BNF 2017).

Patient counselling	• ***Side-effects*** • ***Risk of breathing problems in asthmatic and patients with COPD*** • ***Risk of hypoglycaemia in diabetics*** • ***Compliance*** • ***Withdrawal*** • ***Overdose***	→ Discuss common side-effects of beta blockers. This includes informing male patients that erectile dysfunction may be a side-effect. → If prescribed to patients with obstructive airways disease (this is strongly discouraged), inform patient to call an ambulance if breathing difficulties occur. → If prescribed to diabetic patients, warn them that their beta blocker might mask signs of hypoglycaemia. → Emphasize that patient should not stop taking their beta blocker unless advised by their doctor (British Heart Foundation, *Medicines for your Heart*, 2014). If a patient has been taking beta blockers, it is likely that their body is used to this drug and when they stop taking it they may suffer from 'rebound' symptoms such as worsening of chest pain or arrhythmias. → If beta blockers need to be stopped, normally a dose reduction is undertaken over 7–14 days and it is important that withdrawal is supervised. → The adverse effects of a beta blocker overdose are unpredictable and can be dangerous; hence medical help should be sought immediately.

Calcium channel blockers (CCBs)

Examples	• Non-rate-limiting: amlodipine, felodipine, nifedipine • Rate-limiting: verapamil, diltiazem Note that diltiazem should be prescribed by brand	→ End in -dipine; are also known as dihydropyridine CCBs → Rate-limiting CCBs do not have a common suffix
Mode of action	• Inhibit influx of Ca^{2+} ions into vascular smooth muscle (decrease in intracellular Ca^{2+})	→ Reduces contractility, conductivity and oxygen demand of heart
Routes of delivery	• PO, IV (verapamil and nicardipine)	→ Some CCBs have short $t_{1/2}$ and are available as modified release (MR) preparations.
Indications	• Non-rate-limiting: – Prophylaxis of stable angina – Hypertension • Rate-limiting: same as above – Supraventricular tachycardia – Prophylaxis and treatment of angina – Hypertension Note that diltiazem cream can be used for haemorrhoids	→ 1st line in those who are >55 or Afro-Caribbean (as low-renin hypertension, for which CCBs are effective, is common in this ethnic group) (NICE 2011, CG127) • Mnemonic **ASH (CCB indications)** **A**ngina **S**VT **H**ypertension
Cautions and contraindications	• Unstable angina • Severe aortic stenosis • Recent MI (within 1 month)	
Interactions	• Other antihypertensive drugs e.g. beta blockers • Digoxin • Theophylline • Anti-epileptic drugs	→ Increased hypotensive effect → Increased plasma digoxin concentration → Increased plasma theophylline concentration → Reduced effect of dihydropyridine CCBs
Monitoring	• Determined on an individual basis	→ May include BP measurement or ECG
Side-effects	• Common: – Headache, flushing, abdominal pain, hypotension, tachycardia, fatigue, peripheral oedema and cold peripheries • Less common: – Bradycardia, heart block and heart failure in patients with poor LV function – Impotence (felodipine)	→ Side-effects such as flushing, hypotension, dizziness and ankle swelling may settle down after a couple of weeks and then resolve (British Heart Foundation, *Medicines for Your Heart*, 2014)
Patient counselling	• ***Lifestyle measures:*** discuss reduction of other cardiovascular risk factors e.g. smoking cessation. • ***Food interactions:*** do not consume grapefruit or its juice as this may interact with the drug. • ***Compliance in angina:*** if you have angina and stop taking your CCB, your chest pain might worsen.	→ Grapefruit inhibits the CYP3A4 system, which increases the bioavailability of the calcium channel blocker and potentiates its antihypertensive effects

Cardiac glycosides

Examples	• Digoxin	
Mode of action	• Inhibits the Na$^+$/K$^+$-ATPase membrane pump	→ Inhibition of Na$^+$/K$^+$-ATPase pump causes an increase in intracellular Na$^+$, which is exchanged with extracellular Ca^{2+}. Intracellular Ca^{2+} increases, resulting in an increase in the force of myocardial contraction and a reduction in conductivity in the AV node
Routes of delivery	• PO, IV (IV administration must be slow)	→ When switching from IV to oral route, the dose may need to be increased by 20–33% to maintain the same effect (BNF 2017)
Indications	• Heart failure • Atrial fibrillation and atrial flutter	
Cautions and contraindications	• Patients with heart block, Wolff–Parkinson–White syndrome (WPW), ventricular tachycardia, ventricular fibrillation, myocarditis and cardiomyopathy • Use with caution in hypoxia, hypokalaemia, hypomagnesaemia and hypercalcaemia	→ Associated with increased risk of digoxin toxicity

Interactions	• Drugs that increase risk of digoxin toxicity:
	  – Loop and thiazide diuretics and spironolactone
	  – Calcium channel blockers, amiodarone
	  – Quinine	

Monitoring	• Plasma digoxin level (routinely taken 6 hours post dose, unless toxicity suspected) • Target plasma digoxin level should be 1–2 microgram/L • U+Es and eGFR • Heart rate	→ Obtain a plasma digoxin level as soon as toxicity is suspected → Patients with renal failure require a lower dose of digoxin → Electrolyte disturbances may increase toxicity risk (see Cautions and contraindications) → HR should remain above 60 bpm on maintenance dose

Side-effects	• Common:
	  – GI disturbances, dizziness, nausea, vomiting, blurred or yellowed vision, rash
	• Less common:
	  – Anorexia, depression, gynaecomastia
	• Beware of digoxin toxicity – digoxin has a narrow therapeutic index; however, digoxin toxicity can occur at normal levels
		• Mnemonic **ABCDEF (digoxin toxicity signs)**
		Arrhythmias & **A**nxiety
		Blurred vision
		Confusion
		Dizziness and **D**iarrhoea
		Emesis
		Feeling nauseous

Patient counselling	• ***Digoxin toxicity:*** explain side-effects and signs of digoxin toxicity, and warn patient to seek medical help immediately if signs of digoxin toxicity occur.	→ Digoxin toxicity symptoms: nausea, vomiting, diarrhoea, confusion and blurred vision

Nitrates

Examples	• Glyceryl trinitrate (GTN), isosorbide mononitrate (ISMN), isosorbide dinitrate (ISDN)	→ End in -nitrate
Mode of action	• GTN is converted to nitric oxide (NO)	→ NO causes blood vessels to relax and dilate, there is a reduction in vascular resistance and more blood is delivered to the body; thus angina is relieved by GTN use
Routes of delivery	• Sublingual (tablet or spray), continuous IV infusion, transdermal patch or (rarely) ointment	→ Check if patient has taken GTN at home if presenting with chest pain
Indications	• Treatment of angina (GTN) • Prophylaxis of angina (ISMN and ISDN)	
Cautions and contraindications	• Contraindicated in severe aortic stenosis	→ Vasodilatation by nitrate can cause significant drop in blood pressure – dangerous in fixed cardiac output states
Interactions	• Phosphodiesterase inhibitors (e.g. sildenafil)	
Monitoring	• BP should be monitored when GTN is given as an IV infusion, and systolic BP should not be allowed to fall below 90 mmHg	→ GTN infusion must be stopped if SBP <90 mmHg (unless advised otherwise)

Side-effects	• Common:
	  – Due to vasodilatation: flushing, tachycardia, throbbing headaches, dizziness and postural hypotension*
	• Less common:
	  – Nausea
	  – Syncope
	  – Tolerance may develop after prolonged use of nitrates
	
	*Postural hypotension is defined as abnormal fall in blood pressure of at least 20 mmHg systolic and 10 mmHg diastolic within 3 mins of standing upright.
		• Mnemonic **GTN HEADACHES (nitrate side-effects)**
		Gravity-induced BP drop (postural hypotension)
		Tolerance
		Nausea
		HEADACHES

Patient counselling	• **Demonstrate GTN spray use:** show patient how to take GTN spray and advise patient to take GTN spray with them when they are away from home. • **Take GTN if chest pain occurs:** advise patient to take GTN if chest pain symptoms develop and to ring for an ambulance immediately. • **Side-effects:** warn patient of headaches and postural hypotension when starting treatment. • **Tolerance to nitrates:** may occur after long-term use.	→ Patients who take GTN tablets should be aware that the tablets only last for 8 weeks after opening the bottle

Lipid-regulating drugs (statins)

Examples	• Atorvastatin, pravastatin, rosuvastatin, simvastatin	→ End in -statin
Mode of action	• Inhibit HMG CoA reductase (an enzyme involved in cholesterol production)	→ Lower serum cholesterol levels due to reduced production and increased liver clearance, and cause an increase in HDL cholesterol (the more favourable type of cholesterol)
Routes of delivery	• PO	→ Some statins work better in the evening, whereas others can be taken at any time (British Heart Foundation, *Medicines for Your Heart*, 2014)
Indications	• Primary prevention of CVD • Secondary prevention of CVD • Hypercholesterolaemia (familial or acquired)	→ Statins are the most commonly prescribed type of drug in the UK (British Heart Foundation, *Medicines for Your Heart*, 2014) → One of the five drugs indicated post-MI (NICE 2013, CG172)
Cautions and contraindications	• Pregnant or breastfeeding women • Be careful in renal or hepatic impairment • Use with caution in patients with a high alcohol intake	→ Discontinue 3 months prior to conception – risk of congenital anomalies → Prescribe lower doses in renal or hepatic impairment → Increased risk of hepatic damage
Interactions	• CYP450 inhibitors • Clarithromycin • Amlodipine (simvastatin only) • Concomitant use of fusidic acid and use within 7 days after last dose of fusidic acid • Grapefruit and its juice	→ Statin should be withheld during clarithromycin course → Dose adjustment of simvastatin may be required, as the maximum dose of simvastatin that can be taken alongside amlodipine is 20 mg → Risk of fatal rhabdomyolysis → Simvastatin and atorvastatin are known to interact with these
Monitoring	• Check baseline lipids before starting statins • Check TFTs before starting statins • Check LFTs after 3 months of therapy and after 1 year	→ To monitor clinical effect of statin therapy → Hypothyroidism is a reversible cause of hyperlipidaemia → To look for decline in hepatic function (stop statin if serum transaminases are 3x the upper limit of the normal value)

Side-effects	• Common:
	  – Headache
	  – GI disturbances
	  – Mild muscle aches to severe muscle toxicity
	  – Rise in serum liver enzymes, especially ALT
	• Rare:
	  – Rhabdomyolysis
		• Mnemonic **HMG CoA (statin side-effects)**
		Headache & **H**epatotoxicity
		Myalgia
		GI disturbances
		Complains of rust-coloured urine (rhabdomyolysis)
		Overproduction of serum liver enzymes
		ALT rise (in particular)

Patient counselling	• ***Side-effects and rhabdomyolysis:*** although statins are well tolerated by most people, side-effects should be explained to all patients. Tell patient to report any muscle symptoms to their GP. Warn patient to seek medical help urgently if they have rust-coloured urine. • ***Alcohol:*** advise patients to keep alcohol intake low.	→ Check creatine kinase (CK) if patient describes severe muscle pain, weakness or myoglobinuria and you suspect rhabdomyolysis → Excessive alcohol intake damages the liver and increases the risk of muscle toxicity with statin use

Coumarins		
Examples	• Warfarin	
Mode of action	• It is a vitamin K antagonist and it interferes with the vitamin K cycle by inhibiting enzyme vitamin K epoxide reductase	→ Vitamin K is needed to form clotting factors; hence the use of warfarin reduces the likelihood of clot formation
Route of delivery	• PO	→ Available in different colours representing different strengths: – Brown = 1 mg – Blue = 3 mg – Not commonly used because of risk of medication errors (by a factor of ten!) if mixed up: white (0.5 mg) and pink (5 mg)
Indications	• Prophylaxis and treatment of DVT and PE	→ Duration of treatment variable; dependent on how many times patient has had DVT/PE and whether DVT/PE was spontaneous or provoked; consult local guidelines for more information
	• Prophylaxis of embolism in prosthetic valve	→ Lifelong treatment with warfarin
	• Atrial fibrillation	→ Lifelong treatment with warfarin to prevent TIA and stroke
Cautions and contraindications	• Patients already on anticoagulants	→ Ensure that patient is not taking enoxaparin, apixaban, rivaroxaban, dabigatran or edoxaban → Note that patients are normally given enoxaparin for the first few days of warfarin initiation as it takes warfarin some time to start working
	• Patients on blood thinning agents e.g. aspirin • Patients at high risk of bleeding e.g. haemophiliacs • Recent head injury or haemorrhagic stroke • Pregnant women (dangerous in 1st and 3rd trimesters)	→ Patient safety tip: if the prescriber does not recognize a drug that the patient is taking, it is advisable that the prescriber reviews the drug to ensure that it is compatible with taking warfarin → Teratogenic: effects include facial deformities, cardiac defects, blindness and mental retardation
	• Monitor INR more frequently in severe renal impairment • Avoid in severe hepatic impairment • Caution in uncontrolled hypertension	→ Patients with liver disease may have coagulopathies
Monitoring	• INR will be monitored by GP by a finger prick blood test	→ INR (international normalized ratio) is a measure of how likely the patient's blood is to clot
	• Initially patient will have a blood test every day for 1 week, then once a week until INR at a satisfactory level and after that every 3 months	→ Each patient will have an INR level which is appropriate for them, but normally INR should be maintained between 2.5 and 3.5
Interactions	• Food: vitamin K-containing foods (leafy green vegetables, liver), grapefruit, cranberries (British Heart Foundation, *Medicines for your Heart*, 2014) • Drink: grapefruit juice, cranberry juice, alcohol • Medications: certain types of antibiotics (e.g. macrolides), amiodarone, antidepressants, oral contraceptive pill (reduces efficacy of warfarin), carbamazepine • Smoking • Herbal remedies (St John's wort)	• Mnemonic **The 7 As (main warfarin interactions)** **A**ntibiotics **A**nalgesics **A**ntiplatelet drugs **A**lcohol **A**ntidepressants **A**nti-pregnancy (oral contraceptive pills) **A**miodarone

Coumarins – *cont'd*

Side-effects	• Common: 　– Bleeding and bruising 　– Rash 　– Diarrhoea • Less common: 　– Hypersensitivity reaction to warfarin 　– Warfarin-induced skin necrosis 　– Alopecia (frequency not known)	

Patient counselling	• ***Mode of action and side-effects:*** explain that warfarin thins the blood and may cause bleeding and bruising. If bleeding is excessive, e.g. if the patient suffers from nosebleeds that do not stop, if there is blood in the urine or in the stool or the patient notices severe bruising, they should attend A&E immediately.	
	• ***Yellow Book and heparin:*** when a patient is started on warfarin, they will have to take heparin for a couple of days and they will receive a Yellow Book to bring to appointments to record their INR results and warfarin prescriptions.	➤ Heparin is given by subcutaneous injection and it will only be administered at the start of warfarin treatment (warfarin takes a couple of days to start working) ➤ Emphasize the importance of bringing Yellow Book to appointments
	• ***How to take warfarin and missed doses:*** warfarin should be taken once a day, at the same time every day. It is important not to miss warfarin doses. If a dose is missed, it is advisable that the patient contacts their GP or anticoagulation clinic for advice.	➤ Depending on how late the missed dose is, the patient may be advised to take the missed dose or to omit the missed dose. A patient should never take a double dose if more than 24 hours have passed since a missed dose.
	• ***Food and drug interactions:*** a balanced diet should be maintained when taking warfarin. Avoid excessive amounts of leafy green vegetables and alcohol. Over-the-counter NSAIDs and aspirin should not be taken when taking this drug, and warfarin interacts with many medications and herbal remedies, so check with a doctor or pharmacist before starting a drug.	
	• ***Pregnancy:*** if patient becomes pregnant they must stop taking warfarin immediately.	
	• ***Inform health professionals about warfarin:*** if the patient is having a medical or dental procedure, they should inform their clinician that they are on warfarin.	
	• ***Emergencies:*** attend A&E urgently in cases of head injury.	➤ It is useful to wear a medical alert bracelet to inform others of warfarin use in the case of an emergency
	• ***Contact sports:*** contact sports and other high-risk activities should be avoided whilst on warfarin due to the increased risk of bleeding in the event of minor injury or trauma.	

Factor XA inhibitors (referred to as NOACs – novel oral anticoagulants, or DOACs – direct oral anticoagulants)

Examples	• Apixaban, dabigatran, edoxaban and rivaroxaban	➤ Formerly known as novel oral anticoagulants (NOACs)
Mode of action	• Directly inhibit factor Xa, thus disrupting the clotting cascade	➤ The clotting cascade is dependent on factor Xa
Routes of delivery	• PO	
Indications	• Treatment and prophylaxis of DVT and PE in hip and knee replacements • Stroke prophylaxis in non-valvular AF	
Cautions and contraindications	• Active bleeding or significant risk of major bleeding • Postoperative analgesia with epidural catheter *in situ* • Haemodynamically unstable patients with PE or patients who may undergo thrombolysis or pulmonary embolectomy • Avoid in hepatic impairment, pregnancy and breastfeeding or if creatinine clearance <15 ml/min • Use with caution in patients with prosthetic heart valves	➤ Risk of paralysis, seek expert help
Interactions	• Other anticoagulants	➤ NOACs should never be prescribed to patients who are taking other anticoagulants due to the increased risk of bleeding
Monitoring	• No need for INR monitoring • Monitor patient for signs of bleeding or anaemia • Check eGFR before and after starting treatment	➤ Stop NOAC if severe bleeding occurs ➤ To ensure that baseline renal function is sufficient for drug and to monitor for future renal impairment

Side-effects	• Common:
	  – Bleeding and bruising
	  – GI upset, particularly nausea
	• Less common:
	  – Hepatobiliary disorders (rare in dabigatran use)	

Patient counselling	• ***Compliance:*** emphasize the importance of taking drug as directed. Tablets should be swallowed whole and taken at the same time each day. • ***Concurrent medications:*** the patient should not start any medications without consulting a doctor or pharmacist. • ***Excessive bleeding:*** warn patient to seek medical help urgently if they experience excessive bleeding or bruising. • ***Medical alert bracelet:*** wear a medical alert bracelet.	• Mnemonic **NOAC (NOAC characteristics)** **N**o INR monitoring **O**nly interacts with a few foods and meds **A**void in severe renal impairment **C**an't be readily reversed* *At the time of writing, only rivaroxaban has a licensed reversal agent

Low molecular weight heparins

Examples	• Enoxaparin	→ End in -parin
Mode of action	• Bind to anti-thrombin to form a complex which inactivates clotting factor Xa	→ This prevents clot formation and reduces VTE risk
Route of delivery	• S/C	
Indications	• Prophylaxis and treatment of VTE and PE • MI and unstable ACS	
Cautions and contraindications	• Thrombocytopenia • Anticoagulant use • Patients with renal impairment require dose adjustment • Use with caution in elderly patients, patients with hepatic impairment or low body weight	
Monitoring	• Measure FBC (platelets) and U+Es (serum K$^+$) before starting treatment. • Calculate creatinine clearance to ensure patient's renal function is appropriate for the dose they will be prescribed. If patient's creatinine clearance <30 ml/min, they should be prescribed a halved dose of enoxaparin. • Review dose if there is a change in the patient's renal function • Discontinue if thrombocytopenia occurs	**How to calculate creatinine clearance (CrCl):** $$CrCl = \frac{(140 - age) \times weight\ (kg)}{Cr} \times 1.04\ (♀)\ or\ 1.23\ (♂)$$ Cr denotes the patient's most recent creatinine value from U+Es → Use 1.04 if female patient or 1.23 if male patient
Interactions	• NSAIDs, anticoagulants, antiplatelet drugs	→ Increased risk of bleeding

Side-effects	• Common:
	  – Haemorrhage
	  – Heparin-induced thrombocytopenia (HIT)
	• Less common:
	  – Hypersensitivity and injection site reactions
	  – Skin necrosis
	  – Enoxaparin-induced hyperkalaemia
	  – Alopecia (rare, but may occur after prolonged use)
		• Mnemonic **LMWH (enoxaparin side-effects)**
		Low platelets
		More bleeding (haemorrhage)
		Weird reactions at injection site
		Hyperkalaemia, **H**ypersensitivity and **H**air loss

Patient counselling	• ***Indication and duration:*** explain why patient should take enoxaparin and for how long. • ***Injection technique:*** teach patient how to self-inject enoxaparin and emphasize rotation of injection sites. • ***Excessive bleeding:*** warn patient to seek medical help urgently if excessive bleeding occurs.	→ Enoxaparin is used temporarily during the first couple of days of warfarin therapy, before warfarin starts to work → Enoxaparin is normally injected into the abdomen

Irreversible COX inhibitors

Examples	• Aspirin	
Mode of action	• Irreversibly inhibit COX (non-selective) • Irreversibly inhibit thromboxane A$_2$	➤ COX is involved in prostaglandin release ➤ Thromboxane A$_2$ is needed for platelet aggregation, hence inhibition of thromboxane A$_2$ prevents blood from clotting and forming thrombi
Route of delivery	• PO	
Indications	• Treatment of MI • Prophylaxis of MI (usually taken as 75 mg OD) • Pregnant women at high risk of pre-eclampsia	➤ Usually given as 300 mg aspirin STAT dose ➤ One of the five drugs indicated post-MI (NICE 2013, CG172) ➤ Can be taken from week 12 to delivery in pregnant women at high risk of pre-eclampsia
Cautions and contraindications	• Patients on antiplatelet drugs e.g. clopidogrel • Patients at high risk of bleeding e.g. haemophiliacs • Peptic ulceration • Known hypersensitivity to aspirin or NSAIDs • Children under 16 • Use with caution in patients with asthma or anaemia and in elderly patients • Use with caution during the 3rd trimester of pregnancy	
Monitoring	• Take note of any side-effects when reviewing patient	
Interactions	• NSAIDs, anticoagulants and SSRIs	➤ Increased risk of bleeding
Side-effects	• Frequency not known for the following side-effects: – Aspirin may induce bronchospasm in asthmatics (Samter's triad) – Peptic ulceration (PPI may be co-prescribed to patients at high risk of peptic ulceration) – GI bleeding – Associations with tinnitus and nasal polyps exist (this applies to analgesic doses, which may be higher than the dose used for secondary prevention of cardiac events)	• Mnemonic **ASPIRIN (aspirin side-effects)** **A**sthma **S**alicylism **P**eptic ulcer and **P**remature closure of ductus arteriosus **I**ntestinal blood loss **R**eye's syndrome (in children) **I**ndigestion **N**oise (tinnitus)
Patient counselling	• *How to take aspirin:* • *Prolonged bleeding:* • *Not for children:*	➤ Non-dispersible aspirin should not be chewed. It should be swallowed whole with food and indigestion remedies should be avoided at the time of aspirin consumption. ➤ Aspirin may cause a patient to bleed more or to bleed longer if they sustain an injury. Such symptoms should be reported to the patient's GP. ➤ Do not give to children under the age of 16 (due to risk of causing Reye's syndrome).

Antiplatelet drugs

Examples	• Clopidogrel, ticagrelor	
Mode of action	• Inhibits ADP pathway by binding to PSY_{12} receptors on platelet cell membranes	→ ADP pathway is needed for platelet activation and subsequent platelet aggregation
Routes of delivery	• PO	
Indications	• Primary prevention of cardioembolic events following ACS • Secondary prevention of cardioembolic events following ACS • Clopidogrel or ticagrelor administered prior to coronary stenting procedures • To be taken for one year following coronary procedures	→ 300 mg clopidogrel normally prescribed to patient, with aspirin → Ticagrelor co-prescribed with low-dose aspirin → Can be taken longer than 1 year if decided by medical team
Cautions and contraindications	• Active bleeding • History of intracranial haemorrhage • Pregnancy and breastfeeding • Use with caution in hepatic and renal impairment (avoid if severe)	
Interactions	• Other antiplatelet drugs, anticoagulants, NSAIDs, fibrinolytics, SSRIs • Ulcer healing drugs • Grapefruit juice	→ Increased risk of bleeding → Reduced antiplatelet effect → Grapefruit juice decreases efficacy of clopidogrel – manufacturer advises to avoid (BNF, 2017)
Monitoring	• Monitor patient for side-effects during review appointments • Monitor patient's renal function 1 month after starting ticagrelor	

Side-effects	• Common:
	  – Abdominal pain
	  – Bleeding
	  – Diarrhoea
	• Less common:
	  – Nausea
	  – Vomiting
	  – Gastritis, peptic and duodenal ulceration
	  – Constipation and flatulence
		• Mnemonic **ADP (ADP receptor inhibitor side-effects)**
		Abnormal bleeding
		Diarrhoea and other GI problems
		Peptic and duodenal ulcers

Patient counselling	• **Side-effects:** • **Inform health professionals about drug:** • **Stop before surgery:** • **Pregnancy and breastfeeding:**	→ Explain that drug may cause a patient to bleed longer if they have an injury and that they should seek medical help if they experience severe prolonged bleeding after injury. → If the patient is undergoing a procedure they should inform the responsible clinician about taking antiplatelet drug. → Clopidogrel is normally discontinued 7 days before surgery. → Advice from manufacturers is to avoid clopidogrel in pregnancy and breastfeeding.

Iron supplements

Examples	• Ferrous sulphate, ferrous fumarate	
Mode of action	• Iron supplementation increases the iron stores contained in the body	→ Iron is needed for erythropoiesis and haemoglobin synthesis. If iron deficiency is present, anaemia and symptoms of reduced oxygen-carrying capacity (e.g. shortness of breath) can occur.
Route of delivery	• PO, IV infusion (specialist use only)	→ Iron can be given as an IV infusion; however, this is reserved for specialist use only where patients are acutely unwell → Allergic reactions are common with the parenteral route
Indications	• Treatment and prophylaxis of iron deficiency anaemia	→ Confirm that iron deficiency is the cause of anaemia as there is a risk of iron overload if patients with sufficient iron stores are treated with supplementary iron
Cautions and contraindications	• Peptic ulceration • Known hypersensitivity to aspirin or NSAIDs • Avoid in patients with strictures or diverticula	
Monitoring	• Take note of any side-effects when reviewing patient	
Interactions	• Quinolones, tetracyclines, penicillamine, levodopa	→ Reduced absorption of these drugs when taking oral iron because the iron salts form chelates with the drugs stated

Side-effects	• Common:
	   – GI disturbances (particularly constipation)
	   – Black and tarry stools
		• Mnemonic **Great Britain i.e. GB (iron side-effects)**
		 GI upset
		 Black tarry stools

Patient counselling	• *Side-effects:*	→ Explain that common side-effects of iron therapy are nausea and gastrointestinal disturbances such as diarrhoea, constipation and epigastric pain. Iron tablets can be taken with food to reduce GI disturbances.
	• *Black and tarry stools:*	→ Warn the patient that oral iron may cause black and tarry stools and reassure the patient not to worry if this occurs after commencing treatment.
	• *Taking vitamin C with iron:*	→ Advise the patient that taking ascorbic acid (vitamin C) can help increase the uptake of iron. Hence, the patient may wish to consider taking vitamin C supplements in conjunction with iron tablets, to increase efficacy of treatment.
	• *Compliance before colonoscopy:*	→ If the patient is having a colonoscopy, iron supplements may need to be stopped in advance of procedure for visualization purposes (easier to see during colonoscopy if stools are not black and tarry). Time to stop iron supplements before colonoscopy is normally one week; however, specific advice should be sought from team performing procedure.
	• *Keep iron tablets away from kids:*	→ Ensure that iron tablets are kept out of reach of children as iron poisoning can be fatal.

Corticosteroids (inhaled and systemic glucocorticoids)

Examples	• Inhaled: beclomethasone, budesonide, fluticasone • Systemic (oral and IV): prednisolone, dexamethasone, hydrocortisone	→ Note that these examples of corticosteroids have been listed by their most common route of delivery but some can be administered via other routes
Mode of action	• Bind to steroid receptors and mimic the action of cortisol (endogenous) • Reduce inflammation by causing upregulation of anti-inflammatory mediators	→ Effect on respiratory system: dilates airway and reduces mucosal inflammation and mucus production
Route of delivery	• PO, IV, inhaled or nebulized, topical application	
Indications	• Management of obstructive airways disease (inhaled) • Exacerbation of asthma or COPD (systemic) • Anaphylaxis • Suppression of inflammatory and allergic disease • Inflammatory bowel disease • Nasal polyps	→ IV hydrocortisone used → Steroid nasal sprays can help to shrink nasal polyps
Cautions and contraindications	• Systemic steroids are contraindicated in pregnancy, but inhaled steroids can be taken as normal in pregnancy and breastfeeding • Live vaccines in patients receiving immunosuppressive doses of systemic steroids	→ Risk of intrauterine growth restriction
Monitoring	• Inhaled: monitor asthma or COPD • Systemic: BP measurement and blood glucose prior to treatment and intermittently throughout treatment	→ To monitor cardiovascular and metabolic effects of steroids
Interactions	• NSAIDs • Anti-hypertensives • Anti-diabetic drugs • Warfarin	→ Increased risk of peptic ulceration and bleeding → Reduced hypotensive effect → Steroids antagonize the anti-diabetic effects of these medications → Steroids can increase or decrease anticoagulant effect

Side-effects	• Inhaled corticosteroids:
	  – Oral candidiasis (thrush)
	  – Voice hoarseness
	  – Growth suppression in children
	• Systemic corticosteroids
	• Patients on long-term steroids require osteoporosis prophylaxis (co-prescription of bisphosphonates) and prophylaxis against gastric ulceration (co-prescription of a PPI)
	• Central serous chorioretinopathy is a retinal disorder that has been linked to the systemic use of corticosteroids. Recently, it has also been reported after local administration of corticosteroids via inhaled and intranasal, epidural, intra-articular, topical dermal, and periocular routes.
		• Mnemonic **CORTICOSTEROIDS (steroid side-effects)**
		Cushing's syndrome
		Osteoporosis
		Retardation of growth
		→ **T**hin skin, easy bruising
		Immunosuppression
		Cataracts and glaucoma
		Oedema

Side-effects – **cont'd**	The MHRA recommends that patients should be advised to report any blurred vision or other visual disturbances with corticosteroid treatment given by any route; consider referral to an ophthalmologist for evaluation of possible causes if a patient presents with vision problems (MHRA/CHM advice, August 2017).	**S**uppression of HPA axis **T**runcal obesity **E**motional disturbances **R**ise in BP **O**esophageal and peptic ulceration **I**ncreased hair growth (hirsutism) **D**iabetes mellitus **S**triae Please note that this mnemonic summarizes the main side-effects for all types of corticosteroids, but not all of them apply to each type
Patient counselling	**INHALED CORTICOSTEROIDS** • **In-depth counselling about full side-effects:** if prescribing inhaled corticosteroids, explain common side-effects and discuss risks (including cardiovascular, metabolic and psychological changes) and benefits of treatment. Ask patients to report any visual changes (see previous page). • **Inhaler technique:** educate patient on appropriate inhaler technique and review inhaler technique at follow-up. Consider prescribing a spacer device or breath-actuated inhaler if it is the first time the patient is being prescribed an inhaler or the patient is struggling with using their inhaler. • **Indication for each inhaler:** ensure that the patient knows when to use each type of inhaler if prescribed multiple inhalers i.e. preventer and reliever therapy. • **Preventing oral thrush:** warn patient to gargle with water after using inhaler to prevent oral candidiasis. **SYSTEMIC CORTICOSTEROIDS** • **In-depth counselling about full side-effects:** if prescribing systemic corticosteroids, explain common side-effects and discuss risks (including cardiovascular, metabolic and psychological changes) and benefits of treatment. Ask patients to report any visual changes (see previous page). • **PPI and bisphosphonates:** explain the reason for co-prescribing bisphosphonates and a PPI and emphasize the importance of compliance to avoid adverse effects of long-term steroid treatment. • **Compliance and withdrawal:** it is important that the patient does not stop taking the steroids unless advised by their doctor. Withdrawal of steroids must occur gradually and this should be determined on a case-by-case basis. • **Steroid treatment card:** patient should be given a steroid treatment card to carry. This contains details of prescriber, drug, dose and duration. • **Sick day rules:** ensure patient is aware of sick day rules for steroids (see next page)	• Mnemonic **CUSHINGOID (steroid side-effects)** **C**ataracts **U**lcers **S**triae & **S**kin thinning **H**ypertension **I**mmunosuppression **N**ecrosis (AVN of femoral head) **G**rowth inhibited in children **O**besity & **O**steoporosis **I**ncreased hair growth (hirsutism) **D**iabetes → At its worst, abrupt withdrawal can cause adrenal insufficiency, hypotension or death

Sick day rules for corticosteroids:

- "All patients and their partners should receive regular crisis prevention training including verification of steroid emergency card/bracelet and instruction on stress-related glucocorticoid dose adjustment.
- Generally, hydrocortisone should be doubled during intercurrent illness, such as a respiratory infection with fever, until clinical recovery. Gastrointestinal infections, a frequent cause of crisis, may require parenteral hydrocortisone administration.
- Preferably all patients, but at least patients traveling or living in areas with limited access to acute medical care, should receive a hydrocortisone emergency self-injection kit.
- For major surgery, trauma, delivery, and diseases requiring intensive care unit monitoring, patients should receive IV administration."

(from *J. Clin. Endocrinol. Metab.* 2009;94(4): 1059–1067)

Beta-2 adrenoceptor agonists

Examples	• Short-acting beta-2 adrenoceptor agonists (SABA): salbutamol, terbutaline • Long-acting beta-2 adrenoceptor agonists (LABA): salmeterol, formoterol	
Mode of action	• Bind to beta-2 adrenoceptors in bronchial smooth muscle which activates cyclic AMP (cAMP)	➤ Allows relaxation of the bronchial smooth muscle and dilatation of the airways
Route of delivery	• Inhaled, nebulized, PO, IM, S/C or IV	➤ Can be delivered via endotracheal tube
Indications	• Asthma and COPD • Hyperkalaemia (unlicensed indication for salbutamol) • To delay labour in uncomplicated premature labour (initiated and supervised by specialists only)	➤ Salbutamol helps to shift potassium from the extracellular space to the intracellular space, thus reducing serum potassium levels
Cautions and contraindications	• Severe pre-eclampsia • Use with caution in arrhythmias, cardiovascular disease and hypertension; and susceptibility to QT prolongation, diabetes, hyperthyroidism and hypokalaemia	
Monitoring	• Review the patient's asthma or COPD as per local guidelines	
Interactions	• Methyldopa • Loop and thiazide diuretics, theophylline, steroids	➤ Acute hypotension when given with salbutamol infusion ➤ Increased risk of hypokalaemia

Side-effects	• Common:
	  – Fine tremor
	  – Tachycardia
	  – Palpitations
	  – Anxiety
	• Less common:
	  – Hypokalaemia
	  – Pulmonary oedema
	  – Arrhythmias and myocardial ischaemia
		• Mnemonic **FAT MAP (beta-2 agonist side-effects)**
		Fine tremor
		Anxiety
		Tachycardia
		Myocardial ischaemia
		Arrhythmias
		Palpitations and **P**ulmonary oedema

Patient counselling	• *Inhaler technique:* • *Written asthma action plan:* • *Reason for use:* • *Tremor and palpitations:*	➤ Educate patient on appropriate inhaler technique and review inhaler technique at follow-up (BTS/SIGN Asthma Guideline 2016). Consider prescribing a spacer device or breath-actuated inhaler if the patient is struggling. ➤ Every asthmatic patient must receive a written asthma action plan (BTS/SIGN Asthma Guideline 2016), which describes the appropriate course of action if their asthma symptoms worsen or they become severely short of breath. ➤ Clarify that the inhaler containing the SABA (e.g. salbutamol) is the reliever. LABA should not be used during asthma attacks and the prescribed dose should not be exceeded. ➤ Warn patient about fine tremor and palpitations.

Muscarinic antagonists		
Examples	• Short-acting muscarinic antagonists (SAMA): ipratropium bromide • Long-acting muscarinic antagonists (LAMA): tiotropium bromide	
Mode of action	• Compete with acetylcholine (a neurotransmitter) to bind to muscarinic receptors	→ Acetylcholine is involved in generating action potentials and activating the sympathetic and parasympathetic nervous systems
Routes of delivery	• Inhaled, nebulized or intranasal (for rhinitis)	
Indications	• Acute bronchospasm and severe or life-threatening asthma • Management of reversible obstructive airways disease (asthma and COPD) • Rhinorrhoea • Overactive bladder (OAB) and urge incontinence (solifenacin) • CNS depression in anaesthesia (atropine) • Irritable bowel syndrome (mebeverine)	
Cautions and contraindications	• Use with caution in bladder outflow obstruction, paradoxical bronchospasm, prostatic hypertrophy and in patients who are susceptible to angle-closure glaucoma • Additionally, tiotropium bromide should be used with caution in arrhythmias and heart failure requiring hospitalization in the past 12 months or MI within the past 6 months	
Interactions	• Tricyclic antidepressants • Note that interactions do not generally apply to antimuscarinics administered by inhalation	→ Adverse effects more pronounced
Monitoring	• Review adults annually and children 6-monthly	→ Confirm that correct inhaler technique is being used → Ask about symptomatic improvement and side-effects
Side-effects	• Common: – Constipation, diarrhoea and GI motility disorders – Dry mouth and cough – Headache and sinusitis • Less common: – Angle-closure glaucoma, blurred vision, mydriasis – Palpitations, tachycardia, dizziness – Urinary retention • Rare: – Dental caries	• Mnemonic **ABCDE (antimuscarinic side-effects)** **A**norexia **B**lurred vision **C**onfusion and **C**onstipation **D**ry mouth **E**xpulsion of urine stopped (urinary retention) Alternative: **"Can't see, can't pee, can't shit, can't spit"**

Patient counselling	• *Inhaler technique:*	→ Teach the patient correct inhaler technique and review this during follow-up appointments.
	• *Written asthma action plan:*	→ Ensure that patients who are prescribed a muscarinic antagonist for asthma management have a written asthma action plan, which describes the appropriate course of action if their asthma symptoms worsen or they become severely short of breath. Warn patients to seek medical help if they are using increased doses of the drug.
	• *Side-effects:*	→ Warn patients about the antimuscarinic side-effects as they can be unpleasant. Dry mouth also puts the patient at risk of tooth decay, so advise the patient to use sugar-free chewing gum to help keep mouth moist, or to consult their dentist.
	• *When to stop:*	→ Advise patient to stop taking drug if they experience excessive drowsiness and confusion.

Xanthine derivatives

Examples	• Aminophylline, theophylline Note that xanthine derivatives should be prescribed by brand	
Mode of action	• Exert comparable pharmacological effects to caffeine and theobromine, which are substances with similar structure and properties	→ Allow bronchial smooth muscle relaxation → Increase heart rate, contractility and force of contraction
Route of delivery	• PO, IV (too irritant for IM use)	→ Very slow IV injection over at least 20 min
Indications	• Asthma • COPD	
Cautions and contraindications	• Caution in elderly patients, heart failure, arrhythmias and other cardiovascular disease, liver damage, hyperthyroidism, hypokalaemia and viral infections • Avoid breastfeeding for a couple of hours after taking aminophylline	
Monitoring	• Monitor plasma-theophylline concentration 4–6 hours after modified release; target plasma aminophylline should be 10–20 mg/L • Plasma potassium should be monitored in severe asthma	→ To establish whether drug is within therapeutic range (narrow therapeutic index) → Risk of hypokalaemia when multiple medications (beta-2 agonists, steroids) taken for severe asthma
Interactions	• Other xanthine derivatives • Smoking • Beta-2 agonists • Diuretics • Increased risk of seizures with drugs that lower the seizure threshold e.g. quinolones	→ If aminophylline and theophylline are used concomitantly, the patient can suffer from arrhythmias and convulsions → Decreases plasma concentration of drug → Increased risk of hypokalaemia – use with caution in asthmatic patients who may use these medications → Increased risk of hypokalaemia

Side-effects	• Toxicity can occur (narrow therapeutic index)
	• Common:
	  – Nausea
	  – Vomiting
	  – Hypokalaemia (particularly during concomitant treatment with beta-2 agonist, corticosteroids, diuretics or in hypoxia)
	  – Gastric irritation
	  – Tachycardia
	  – Palpitations
	  – Headache
		• Mnemonic **Vomiting Patient Agreed To Have NG Tube (Xanthine derivatives side-effects)**
		Vomiting
		Palpitations
		Arrhythmias
		Tachycardia
		Headache
		Nausea
		Gastric irritation
		Toxicity

Side-effects – **cont'd**	• Rare:
	  – Pulmonary oedema
	  – Arrhythmias
	  – Myocardial ischaemia	

Patient counselling	• ***Toxicity symptoms:*** warn patient about symptoms of toxicity (seizures, hypotension and arrhythmias). • ***Smoking habits:*** remind the patient to inform you if they start or stop smoking during treatment.	→ Dose adjustment may be required if a patient changes their smoking habits

Leukotriene receptor antagonists

Examples	• Montelukast, zafirlukast	→ End in -lukast
Mode of action	• Block the action of cysteinyl leukotrienes in the airways. Cysteinyl leukotrienes are involved in eosinophil or mast cell induced bronchoconstriction.	→ The use of leukotriene receptor antagonist allows bronchodilation
Routes of delivery	• PO	
Indications	• Asthma (chronic) • Allergic rhinitis	
Cautions and contraindications	• Caution in elderly patients and in hepatic impairment (only zafirlukast)	
Interactions	• Warfarin (zafirlukast only)	→ Increased anticoagulant effect
Monitoring	• PEFR measurement will show improvement • Check FBC for agranulocytosis and ask about symptoms suggestive of serious side-effects	

Side-effects	• Common:
	  – Headache
	  – Abdominal pain
	  – Thirst
	• Less common:
	  – Agranulocytosis (zafirlukast only)
	  – Churg–Strauss syndrome
	  – Hypersensitivity
	  – Hepatic disorders
		• Mnemonic **CHAT (leukotriene receptor antagonist side-effects)**
		Churg–Strauss syndrome
		Headache, **H**ypersensitivity and **H**epatic disorders
		Abdominal pain and **A**granulocytosis
		Thirst

Patient counselling	• ***How to take drug:***	→ Can be supplied as tablets or granules. Granules may be swallowed or mixed with cold, soft food (but not fluid) and taken immediately.
	• ***Side-effects, agranulocytosis and Churg–Strauss syndrome:***	→ Inform patient about side-effects of drug. Warn the patient about the signs of agranulocytosis i.e. increased susceptibility to infections (e.g. sore throats), and tell patient to report such occurrences to their GP. Warn the patient about the signs of Churg–Strauss syndrome such as vasculitic rashes, pulmonary problems, cardiac complications and peripheral neuropathy and tell the patient to report these symptoms to their GP.
	• ***Jaundice:***	→ Warn patient to inform their GP if they develop jaundice (yellowing of skin and sclera).
	• ***Angioedema:***	→ If the patient develops breathing difficulties or swelling of tongue or face after taking drug, they should seek medical help urgently.

Antihistamines

Examples	• Non-sedating: cetirizine, fexofenadine, loratadine • Sedating: chlorphenamine, promethazine, cyclizine	→ Cyclizine mainly used to treat nausea and vomiting
Mode of action	• Compete with histamines for binding to the histamine H₁ receptors, thus blocking the effects of the histamine	→ Histamines cause vasodilatation and increased vascular permeability. In anaphylaxis, histamines are released and vasodilatation is widespread and results in significant hypotension.
Route of delivery	• PO, IV (in anaphylaxis)	
Indications	• Emergency treatment of anaphylaxis (chlorphenamine) • Pruritus and urticaria • Seasonal allergic rhinitis • Antiemesis (most common indication for cyclizine) • Insomnia	→ Chlorphenamine is the most effective antihistamine for treating urticaria and pruritus
Cautions and contraindications	• Use with caution in prostatic enlargement, urinary retention, pyloric stenosis, pyloroduodenal obstruction, epilepsy and in patients at risk of angle-closure glaucoma • Check advice from manufacturer before taking a specific antihistamine during pregnancy or breastfeeding	
Monitoring	• Monitor patient for symptomatic improvement • Follow local protocols for post-anaphylaxis monitoring	
Interactions	• Tricyclic antidepressants and MAOIs • Muscarinic antagonists	→ Increased sedation and antimuscarinic effects → Antimuscarinic effects become very pronounced

Side-effects	• Common:
	  – Headache
	  – Drowsiness
	  – Antimuscarinic effects
	• Less common:
	  – Extrapyramidal side-effects
	  – Hypersensitivity reactions
	  – Psychomotor impairment	

Patient counselling	• **Carry antihistamine with you:** advise patients to carry antihistamines with them if they suffer allergic reactions, particularly in cases where specific causative allergens are unknown. If the allergy is severe or the patient has a history of anaphylaxis, the patient should carry an adrenaline auto-injector pen and be trained in its use.	• Mnemonic **DON'T LET YOU FALL ASLEEP (non-sedating antihistamines)** **D**esloratadine **L**oratadine **F**exofenadine **C**etirizine Note that the non-sedating antihistamines are less likely to cause drowsiness but it may still occur

Antihistamines – *cont'd*

Patient counselling – **cont'd**	• **Drowsiness and impairment of function:** warn patient about drowsiness as this may impair the patient's ability to drive or operate machinery. This is not advised when the patient is taking sedating antihistamines and the patient should follow specific instructions from the manufacturer of the antihistamines they are taking regarding driving safety and use of machinery. • **Non-sedating types:** consider prescribing non-sedating antihistamines to patients who need to drive or operate machinery as part of their work, or for patients who have suffered from drowsiness and found this difficult to cope with.	Alternative: **"Non-sedating H₁ blockers keep you a-wake and they end in a-dine"** (**Note:** there are non-sedating antihistamines that are not H₁ blockers; however, this mnemonic is useful for identifying non-sedating H₁ blockers)

Proton pump inhibitors (PPIs)

Examples	• Omeprazole, pantoprazole, lansoprazole, esomeprazole	→ End in -prazole
Mode of action	• Irreversibly inhibit H⁺/K⁺-ATPase in gastric parietal cells, which suppresses gastric acid production	
Route of delivery	• PO, IV	
Indications	• Gastro-oesophageal reflux disease (GORD) • Treatment of gastric and duodenal ulcers • *H. pylori* eradication (triple therapy) • Prophylaxis of ulceration in patients prescribed NSAIDs and corticosteroids • Zollinger–Ellison syndrome	
Cautions and contraindications	• Patients who report 'red flag' symptoms of gastric cancer e.g. weight loss, dysphagia • Caution with patients at risk of osteoporosis • Prescribe lower doses in hepatic impairment	→ Monitor liver function in patients with hepatic impairment
Monitoring	• Exclude gastric malignancy in patients presenting with alarm symptoms before starting drug • Monitor serum magnesium in patients before and during therapy • Enquire about severity of symptoms at review appointments • Endoscopy can be used to visualize ulcers	→ Hypomagnesaemia most frequently occurs after 1 year of taking a PPI but sometimes after only 3 months
Interactions	• Warfarin, clopidogrel (only omeprazole interacts) • Digoxin	→ PPI influences the efficacy of these drugs → Can contribute to hypomagnesaemia

Side-effects	• Common:
	  – GI disturbances
	  – dry mouth
	  – headaches
	  – fatigue
	• Less common
	  – increased likelihood of *Clostridium difficile* infection
	  – increased likelihood of osteoporosis
		• Mnemonic **PPI (PPI side-effects)**
		Pain (headaches, abdominal pain)
		Prone to catch *C. diff* and get osteoporosis
		Intestinal (GI) upset

Patient counselling	• ***Measures to reduce acidity:*** explain that drug reduces acidity of stomach and should hopefully ease symptoms, but advise patient to avoid foods and drinks that exacerbate symptoms, to avoid large meals particularly late in the evening and to avoid lying down immediately after eating. • ***Compliance:*** emphasize the importance of compliance, particularly if this drug has been co-prescribed with other drugs for prophylaxis of ADR. • ***Preventing osteoporosis:*** advise patients who are at risk of osteoporosis to maintain an adequate intake of vitamin D and calcium. • ***Red flags:*** inform patients about 'red flag' symptoms of gastric cancer and tell them to report these to GP.	→ PPIs can 'mask' alarm symptoms of gastric cancer, so it is important to have a high index of suspicion → Consider prophylactic therapy, i.e. bisphosphonates, in cases where patients might struggle to maintain an adequate intake

H₂ receptor antagonists

Examples	• Ranitidine, cimetidine	→ End in -tidine
Mode of action	• Acts on the H₂ receptors to reduce gastric acid production	
Routes of delivery	• PO	
Indications	• Treatment of peptic and duodenal ulcers and GORD	
Cautions and contraindications	• Caution in renal impairment, use halved dose if eGFR <50 ml/min	
Interactions	• Cimetidine interacts with warfarin, phenytoin, theophylline, carbamazepine, sodium valproate • Cimetidine also interacts with clopidogrel	→ Cimetidine is a CYP450 inhibitor, hence it inhibits the metabolism of the aforementioned drugs → Reduced antiplatelet effect of clopidogrel
Monitoring	• Exclude gastric malignancy in patients with alarm symptoms before starting drug	

Side-effects	• Common:
	  – Headache
	  – Dizziness
	  – Diarrhoea
	• Less common:
	  – Rashes
	  – Confusion
	  – Depression
	  – Blood disorders
	  – Gynaecomastia and impotence (cimetidine)
		• Mnemonic **DISCO (drugs that cause gynaecomastia)**
		Digoxin (after long-term use)
		Isoniazid
		Spironolactone
		Cimetidine
		Oestrogens

Patient counselling	• *Reducing acidity:* • *Red flags:*	→ Explain that drug reduces acidity of stomach and should provide symptomatic relief, but advise patient to avoid foods and drinks that worsen symptoms and to avoid large late meals or lying down after eating. → Inform patients about 'red flag' symptoms of gastric cancer and tell them to report these to GP.

Antiemetics

Examples	• H_1 receptor antagonists: cyclizine, promethazine	→ H_1 receptor antagonists block histamine H_1 and acetylcholine receptors in chemoreceptor trigger zone (vomiting centre)
	• Serotonin 5-HT_3-receptor antagonists: ondansetron	→ Precise mode of action for ondansetron not known
	• Dopamine D_2 receptor antagonists: metoclopramide, domperidone, prochlorperazine	→ Dopamine D_2 receptor antagonists inhibit dopaminergic stimulation on the chemoreceptor trigger zone
	• Phenothiazines: prochlorperazine, chlorpromazine	→ Phenothiazines block a variety of receptors that stimulate the chemoreceptor trigger zone, including dopamine, histamine and acetylcholine
	• Muscarinic antagonists: hyoscine	→ Hyoscine exerts a spasmolytic action on the smooth muscle of the gastrointestinal, biliary and genitourinary tracts, and has peripheral anticholinergic effects on the visceral wall
Mode of action	• See above	
Route of delivery	• PO, IV, IM or rectal	

Indications	• Nausea
	• Vomiting:
	  – Drug-induced vomiting (cyclizine)
	  – Vomiting in pregnancy (promethazine)
	  – Postoperative vomiting (hyoscine)
	• Motion sickness (hyoscine)	

Cautions and contraindications	• Avoid phenothiazines in Parkinson's disease and avoid D_2 receptors in young people, particularly females of child-bearing age	→ Increased risk of extrapyramidal side-effects when medications from these drug classes are used
	• Due to its cardiac side-effects, domperidone is contraindicated in people with underlying cardiac conditions, hepatic impairment or taking medications that prolong the QT interval or inhibit the CYP3A4 system (MHRA guidance 2013)	→ To reduce the risk of cardiac side-effects, domperidone is further restricted to use for relief of nausea and vomiting
	• Metoclopramide is associated with severe neurological adverse effects so it should only be used short-term, up to 5 days, and its indications for use have been restricted (MHRA/CHM advice 2013)	→ For further information, review MHRA/CHM guidance and resources
Monitoring	• Enquire about symptoms • ECG (prolonged QT) in patients taking 5-HT_3-receptor antagonists or phenothiazines	

Antiemetics – *cont'd*

Interactions	<ul><li>Where possible, avoid combinations of antiemetics, particularly metoclopramide with ondansetron and metoclopramide or domperidone with cyclizine</li><li>Cyclizine: interacts with opioid analgesics (increased sedative effects) and with anticholinergic drugs</li><li>Ondansetron: interacts with SSRIs and SSRI-related antidepressants and has an enhanced antiemetic action when used with steroids</li><li>Metoclopramide: its action is antagonized by opioid receptor antagonists</li><li>Domperidone: H_2 receptor antagonists and antacids reduce the absorption of domperidone</li><li>Hyoscine: see muscarinic antagonists (p. 22)</li></ul>	
Side-effects	Below are listed important side-effects to be aware of for each type of antiemetic:<ul><li>Drowsiness (H_1 receptor antagonists, phenothiazines)</li><li>Postural hypotension (phenothiazines, muscarinic antagonists)</li><li>Dry mouth (muscarinic antagonists)</li><li>Diarrhoea, constipation and headaches (several types)</li><li>Prolonged QT interval (5-HT_3-receptor antagonists, phenothiazines)</li><li>Extrapyramidal side-effects (D_2 receptor antagonists)</li></ul>	
Patient counselling	<ul><li>***Indication and side-effects:*** explain why you are prescribing an antiemetic and inform the patient about the side-effects of the antiemetic that is being prescribed.</li><li>***Impairment of function:*** warn the patient if the antiemetic may impair their ability to drive or operate machinery, or whether it may put them at higher risk of falls due to dizziness or postural hypotension.</li><li>***Extrapyramidal side-effects:*** if relevant to the antiemetic being prescribed, describe signs of extrapyramidal side-effects to the patient and warn the patient to tell a doctor if these signs occur.</li><li>***Changing antiemetic if no relief:*** tell patient to inform a doctor if their symptoms are not relieved, so that another antiemetic can be used.</li></ul>	→ Extrapyramidal side-effects (EPSE) include *tremor*, *bradykinesia* (slowed movements), *acute dystonia* (involuntary muscular contractions resulting in abnormal posture or balance), *akathisia* (motor restlessness), *tardive dyskinesia* (jerky irregular movements of tongue, face and jaw) and *parkinsonism* (triad of tremor, bradykinesia and rigidity)

Laxatives

Examples	• Stimulant: senna, bisacodyl	→ Increases volume of stool in the colon and stimulates peristalsis
	• Bulk-forming: isphagula husk, methylcellulose	→ Increases stool volume, which makes it easier to pass
	• Osmotic: lactulose, macrogol	→ Increases amount of H_2O in the large bowel
Mode of action	• See above	
Routes of delivery	• PO, PR	→ Avoid rectal route if haemorrhoids or anal fissures are present
Indications	• Constipation	
	• Bowel preparation	
Cautions and contraindications	• Intestinal obstruction	
	• Avoid using osmotic laxatives in patients with fluid overload or electrolyte disturbances	
Interactions	• None	
Monitoring	• Enquire about symptoms	
	• In hospital inpatients, stool charts can be used to monitor and document frequency of bowel motions	→ To inform medical team of improvement of constipation
Side-effects	• Common:	
	– Diarrhoea	
	– Abdominal discomfort	
	– Nausea and vomiting (bisacodyl)	
	• Less common:	
	– Prolonged use of stimulant laxatives can cause an atonic non-functioning colon and hypokalaemia	
Patient counselling	• ***Reason for use and mode of action:***	→ Explain indication and mechanism of action of the prescribed laxative.
	• ***Compliance:***	→ Strongly encourage compliance, particularly in patients taking bowel preparation. Although bowel preparation is unpleasant to take, the more of the bowel preparation the patient takes, the easier it will be for the surgeon to visualize the colon during colonoscopy or surgery.
	• ***Frequency:***	→ Inform patient that they will be making frequent visits to the toilet on this medication.
	• ***Hydration is important:***	→ The patient should aim to drink 6–8 glasses of water each day when taking laxatives.
	• ***Storage:***	→ Bulk-forming laxatives should be kept in a dry environment.

Prescribing in renal impairment:

Which patients are at increased risk of drug-related nephrotoxicity?
- Elderly patients
- Patients with known renal impairment, dehydration, diabetes, heart failure or sepsis

What drugs can cause renal impairment?
- ACE inhibitors and ARBs reduce the GFR by vasodilating the efferent arteriole more than the afferent arteriole.
- NSAIDs inhibit prostaglandin synthesis. Prostaglandins cause vasodilatation of renal arteries, hence NSAIDs decrease renal perfusion. NSAIDs can also cause interstitial nephritis and acute tubular necrosis.
- Diuretics can reduce plasma volume, which in turn reduces renal blood flow.
- Although metformin is not a nephrotoxic drug, the kidneys excrete 90% of the drug. This can put further strain on the kidneys, particularly if underperforming, and metformin can accumulate in patients suffering from renal impairment or AKI, which increases the risk of lactic acidosis. It is important that metformin is not taken within 48 hours of IV receiving contrast as this combination results in a serious nephrotoxic insult to the patient.
- The administration of intravenous contrast can result in contrast-induced nephropathy, which is an acute kidney injury that occurs within 72 hours of receiving IV contrast. It is further defined as an increase in serum creatinine of 25% or by 44 µmol/L from the baseline creatinine value. Contrast-induced nephropathy is reversible, but it is preferable to avoid causing it in the first place. It is advisable to administer IV fluids before and after administration of IV contrast.
- Some types of antibiotics (aminoglycosides, vancomycin, penicillins, amphotericin and sulphonamides) and antivirals (aciclovir) contribute to renal impairment by various mechanisms.
- Some immunosuppressive agents, such as ciclosporin and tacrolimus, are nephrotoxic and they should not be taken concurrently.
- In addition, statins, alcohol and some drugs of abuse (cocaine, heroin, methadone and metamphetamines) have been implicated in causing rhabdomyolysis. Overdoses of paracetamol and aspirin can have an impact on the kidneys, causing acute tubular necrosis and renal papillary necrosis, respectively.

What can be done to prevent renal impairment when prescribing?
- Avoid nephrotoxic drugs in patients at risk of renal impairment.
- If even mild renal impairment is suspected, renal function should be checked before prescribing a new drug.
- Advise patient to drink plenty of fluids, preferably water.
- Give IV fluids before and after the patient experiences a nephrotoxic insult, e.g. IV contrast administration.
- Monitor renal function during therapy, particularly after dose adjustments.
- If renal impairment is confirmed, stop the **DAMN (Diuretics, ACEi/ARBs, Metformin, NSAIDs)** drugs
- If it is essential to prescribe a nephrotoxic drug to manage a condition, the prescriber should consider reducing the dose.

What problems does renal impairment cause in patients?
- Reduced clearance of some drugs or their metabolites, which may accumulate in the body and cause other problems
- Reduced clinical effect of certain drugs in co-existing renal impairment
- Patients with renal impairment may become less tolerant of drug side-effects.

The site of action in the nephron for different types of diuretics

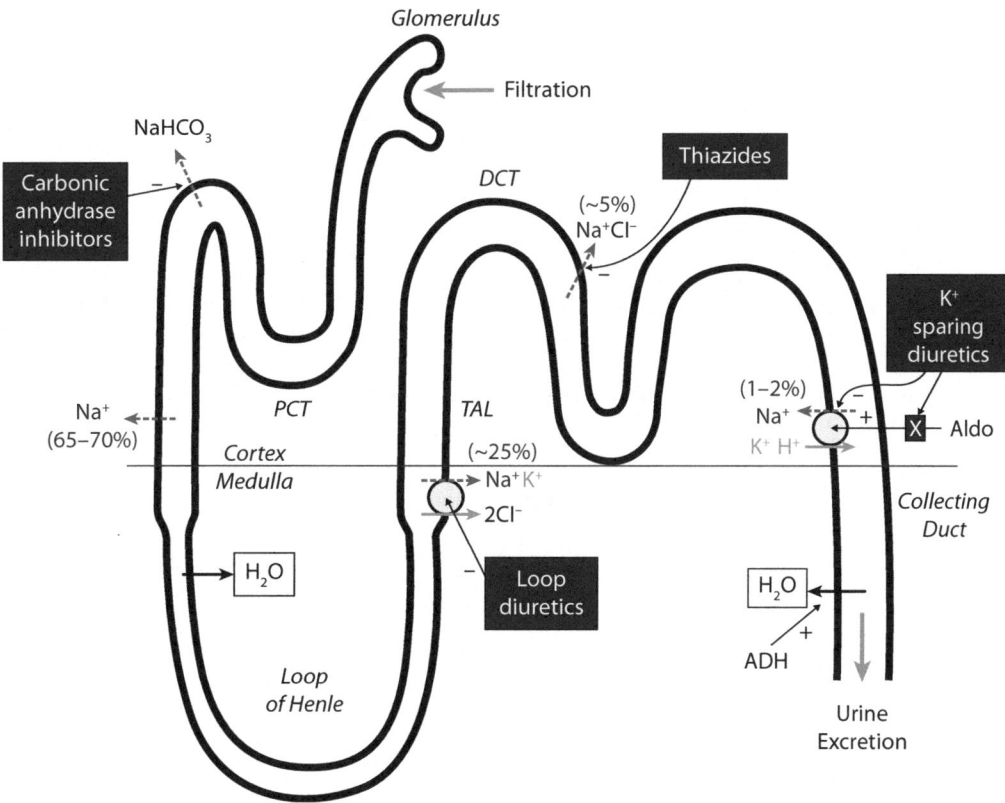

Reproduced with permission from Dr Richard E. Klabunde. Available at www.cvpharmacology.com/diuretic/diuretics

Diuretics

Examples	• Loop diuretics: furosemide, bumetanide	→ Inhibit $Na^+/K^+/2Cl^-$ co-transporter in the loop of Henle
	• Thiazide diuretics: bendroflumethiazide	→ Inhibit Na^+/Cl^- co-transporter in DCT (proximal part), take effect within 1–2 hours and have a duration of action up to 24 hours
	• Aldosterone antagonists (potassium-sparing) diuretics: spironolactone, amiloride	→ Prevent reabsorption of Na^+ in the DCT, thus causing Na^+ and H_2O excretion and K^+ retention
	• Osmotic diuretics: mannitol	→ Cause reabsorption of H_2O in the PCT and the descending limb of the loop of Henle and oppose the action of ADH in the collecting duct
	• Carbonic anhydrase inhibitors: acetazolamide	→ Block carbonic anhydrase at the PCT, so bicarbonate cannot be reabsorbed and is retained in the PCT with H_2O and Na^+
Mode of action	• See above	
Routes of delivery	• PO, IV, topical	
Indications	• Acute pulmonary oedema and chronic heart failure (loop diuretics) • Oliguric renal insufficiency (loop diuretics) • Hypertension (thiazides and thiazide-like diuretics, potassium-sparing diuretics) • Nephrogenic diabetes (thiazides and thiazide-like diuretics) • Hypokalaemia (potassium-sparing diuretics) • Ascites and oedema secondary to hepatic cirrhosis (potassium-sparing diuretics) • Cerebral oedema, raised intraocular pressure and treatment of cystic fibrosis (osmotic diuretics) • Glaucoma (carbonic anhydrase inhibitors)	→ Loop diuretics provide symptomatic improvement but do not reduce mortality in heart failure → The patient must be adequately hydrated before using loop diuretic to produce diuresis

Contraindications	• Diuretics should be used with caution in the elderly, and with the lowest dose possible, because they are particularly susceptible to the side-effects
	• Diuretics should be avoided in pregnancy due to risk of volume depletion
	• Loop diuretics:
	  – Caution in hypovolaemia, hypotension, prostatic hypertrophy and in patients with history of diabetes or gout
	  – Avoid in anuria, severe hyponatraemia, severe hypokalaemia and in comatose or precomatose states associated with liver cirrhosis	

Contraindications – **cont'd**	• Thiazide and thiazide-like diuretics:
	   – Caution in malnutrition, renal impairment and in patients with a history of gout or diabetes
	   – Avoid in Addison's disease, symptomatic hyperuricaemia and in refractory hyponatraemia
	• Potassium-sparing diuretics:
	   – Caution in renal impairment (avoid if severe)
	   – Avoid in hyperkalaemia, hyponatraemia, anuria and Addison's disease
	• Osmotic diuretics:
	   – Use with caution in asthma and haemoptysis, if given by inhaled route
	   – Avoid in anuria, intracranial bleeding except in craniotomy, severe heart failure, severe pulmonary oedema
	   – When given by inhalation, avoid in patients with an impaired lung function or patients who are hyperresponsive to mannitol
	• Carbonic anhydrase inhibitors:
	   – Use with caution in the elderly, diabetic patients, patients with renal calculi and in those with impaired alveolar ventilation
	   – Avoid in adrenocortical insufficiency, hyperchloraemic acidosis, hypokalaemia and hyponatraemia and avoid long-term use in chronic angle-closure glaucoma
		→ Drug can precipitate gout attacks and worsen glycaemic control
		
		→ Thiazide diuretics should not be used to treat gestational hypertension

Interactions	• Interactions common to loop diuretics, thiazides and thiazide-like diuretics and potassium-sparing diuretics:
	   – Drug affecting RAAS system i.e. ACE inhibitors, ARBs, direct renin inhibitors
	   – Anti-hypertensive drugs
	   – NSAIDs
	   – Lithium
	• K^+ supplements should not be taken with potassium-sparing diuretics due to the risk of hyperkalaemia
	• There is a possible increase in nephrotoxicity when mannitol and ciclosporin are taken together
	• There is an increased risk of osteomalacia when carbonic anhydrase inhibitors are used with phenytoin and phenobarbital
	• Acetazolamide increases risk of hypokalaemia when taken with aminophylline and hypokalaemia induced by acetazolamide increases the risk of cardiac toxicity with amiodarone
		→ Increased risk of hyperkalaemia
		
		→ Increased hypotensive effect
		→ Increased risk of nephrotoxicity
		→ Increased risk of lithium toxicity

Monitoring	• Monitor fluid and electrolyte balance and serum osmolality and review cardiac, pulmonary and renal function • Monitor serum potassium level during treatment • Consider measuring daily weights in patients using diuretics for relief of fluid overload	→ Discontinue treatment if hyperkalaemia occurs. If borderline K^+ elevation, request ECG to look for cardiac changes.

Diuretics – *cont'd*	

Side-effects	Below are listed important side-effects to be aware of for each type of diuretic:
	
	• Loop diuretics:
	  – Hypokalaemia
	  – Hyponatraemia
	  – Ototoxicity
	  – Hyperuricaemia
	  – Acute urinary retention
	  – High doses or rapid IV administration of furosemide can cause tinnitus or deafness
	• Thiazides and thiazide-like diuretics:
	  – Hypokalaemia
	  – Altered blood lipids
	  – Postural hypotension
	  – Impotence
	  – May precipitate gout attacks and increase risk of pancreatitis
	• Potassium-sparing diuretics:
	  – GI disturbances
	  – Acute renal failure
	  – Hyperkalaemia
	  – Hyponatraemia
	  – Gynaecomastia
	  – Hypogonadism
	  – Menstrual irregularities in women
	  – Impotence in men
	• Osmotic diuretics:
	  – When inhaled: cough, bronchospasm, wheezing, haemoptysis, irritation and pain in throat, vomiting
	  – When given IV: electrolyte and fluid imbalances, hypotension, thrombophlebitis
	• Carbonic anhydrase inhibitors:
	  – Ataxia
	  – Dizziness
	  – Changes in mood and libido
	  – Nausea
	  – Loss of appetite
	  – Taste disturbance
	  – Thirst

Patient counselling	In addition to explaining the side-effects of the diuretic the patient is being prescribed, mention the following:	
	• *Frequency and nocturia:*	→ Inform patient that the drug will make them pass more urine and it is advisable to take doses during the day to prevent nocturia.
	• *Compliance with monitoring:*	→ Emphasize the importance of blood tests to detect harmful electrolyte imbalances (e.g. hyponatraemia, hypo- or hyperkalaemia) to enable treatment.
	• *Specific to potassium-sparing diuretics:*	→ The patient should take this drug with or after food and they should not take potassium supplements whilst taking this drug. It is not advisable to take NSAIDs, such as ibuprofen, when taking this medication. If the patient becomes unwell with vomiting and diarrhoea, they should stop taking the drug to prevent dehydration and contact their doctor for further management.
	• *Dietary intake of salt:*	→ Advise patients to restrict their intake of salt.

Immunosuppressants

Examples	• Tacrolimus, ciclosporin • Treatment with immunosuppressants should be initiated by specialists • It is important that these drugs are prescribed by brand name and once a patient is stabilized on a particular brand, they should be maintained on this brand to avoid fluctuations in drug serum levels. Specialist help should be sought if it is decided that the patient should be switched brand or immunosuppressant drug.	→ There have been reports of toxicity and graft rejection in cases where brands have been inadvertently switched
Mode of action	• Inhibit calcineurin, which activates T cells to produce an immune response and activates inflammation in the skin	
Routes of delivery	• PO, IV or topical	
Indications	• Prophylaxis against organ rejection in liver, kidney and heart allograft recipients • Allograft rejection resistant to immunosuppressive therapies • Moderate to severe eczema (tacrolimus) • Rheumatoid arthritis (ciclosporin) • Atopic dermatitis and psoriasis (ciclosporin)	
Cautions and contraindications	• Hypersensitivity to macrolides • Pregnancy and breastfeeding • Do not administer tacrolimus and ciclosporin concurrently • Caution in hepatic impairment	→ Tacrolimus is a non-antibiotic macrolide → Risk of premature delivery and intrauterine growth restriction
Interactions	• Grapefruit juice, some types of antibiotics • Aminoglycosides, ibuprofen	→ Increases plasma concentration of tacrolimus → Increased risk of nephrotoxicity
Monitoring	• Monitor BP and ECG (risk of cardiomyopathy) • Monitor LFTs and U+Es (renal function)	

Side-effects	Below are listed important side-effects to be aware of for each type of immunosuppressant:
	• Tacrolimus:
	  – Nephrotoxicity, resulting in acute renal failure
	  – Cardiomyopathy
	  – Glucose metabolism
	  – Increased risk of skin cancer
	• Ciclosporin:
	  – Hypertension
	  – Nephrotoxicity, resulting in acute renal failure
	  – Hepatotoxicity
	  – Gingival hyperplasia
	  – Hyperkalaemia
	  – Hypercholesterolaemia	

Patient counselling	• **Risk of infections:**	→	Explain that the patient is at a higher risk of infections due to immunosuppression and warn the patient to seek medical help if they have a high temperature or feel unwell.
	• **Keep the same brand during treatment:**	→	Make patient aware of the fact that it is important to stay on the same brand of immunosuppressant during treatment (unless advised by senior specialist). By being given this information, the patient will be vigilant to changes in brand and this can prevent unintentional patient safety errors.
	• **Protect your skin from the sun:**	→	As there is an increased risk of skin malignancies when taking certain types of immunosuppressant, it is important to avoid sunbeds and to use suncream and other protective measures.
	• **Impairment of skilled tasks:**	→	Advise patient that these drugs may affect performance of skilled tasks e.g. driving.

Thyroid hormones

Examples	• Levothyroxine	
Mode of action	• Replace low level of thyroxine (T_4) in patients with underactive thyroid glands, which in turn suppresses high TSH levels by negative feedback	➤ This restores a patient's thyroid hormone balance and should stop symptoms of hypothyroidism such as lethargy, tiredness, weight gain and thinning of skin and hair ➤ Beware of over-replacement of thyroxine, characterized by a normal thyroxine level with a low TSH level
Route of delivery	• PO	
Indications	• Primary hypothyroidism • As 'replace' element of 'block and replace' regimen for hyperthyroidism • Goitre • Hashimoto's thyroiditis • Thyroid carcinoma • Hypopituitarism • Thyroid hormones can also be used in pregnancy-related hypothyroidism	
Cautions and contraindications	• Thyrotoxicosis • Use with caution in long-standing hypothyroidism, adrenal insufficiency and in angina and cardiovascular disorders	
Monitoring	• Baseline ECG when starting drug • TFTs should be done 3 months after starting treatment or changing a dose, followed by annual TFTs once patient is stable • Assess maternal thyroid function before conception, at diagnosis of pregnancy, during 2nd and 3rd trimesters and after delivery • Consider supplementation with vitamin D in long-term treatment with levothyroxine	➤ For comparison with future ECGs taken if patients develop cardiovascular side-effects from the thyroid hormone replacement ➤ Levothyroxine dose may need to be increased during pregnancy and if doses are altered, monitoring of thyroid function should be more frequent
Interactions	• Warfarin • Antacids, calcium and iron salts • CYP450 inducers	➤ Enhanced anticoagulant effect ➤ Avoid concurrent use by maintaining a 4-hour gap • Mnemonic **PC BRAS (CYP450 inducers)** **P**henytoin **C**arbamazepine **B**arbiturates **R**ifampicin **A**lcohol (chronic) **S**ulphonylureas

Side-effects	• Common:
	  – GI upset
	  – Palpitations
	  – Tremor
	  – Angina
	  – Goitre
	  – Restlessness
	  – Flushing
	  – Headache
	• Less common:
	  – Angina
	  – Muscular weakness
	  – Weight changes
	  – Insomnia
	  – Mood changes
		• Mnemonic **THYROID (thyroxine side-effects)**
		Tremor
		Heart racing (palpitations)
		"**Y**ou may lose weight rapidly"
		Restlessness
		Out of character (mental or mood changes)
		Insomnia
		Diarrhoea

Patient counselling	• ***Mode of action:*** explain that this medication contains a hormone (thyroxine) that the patient's body is not producing to an adequate level and as a result the patient is experiencing symptoms. • ***How to take:*** it is preferred to take levothyroxine in the morning 30 minutes to 1 hour before having breakfast or taking other medications. • ***Duration of treatment and monitoring:*** inform the patient that treatment is likely to be lifelong and that regular blood tests will be required to monitor thyroid function. • ***Dosing:*** thyroid hormone replacement is normally taken once daily. The patient will be started on the minimum dose and then the dose will be titrated up if required. • ***Compliance:*** it is important that the patient takes the drug as directed and that the patient does not stop taking the drug on his or her own initiative. • ***Signs of thyrotoxicosis:*** warn the patient of the signs of thyrotoxicosis (too much thyroxine) i.e. palpitations, arrhythmias, angina, tremor and diarrhoea. These signs can take up to 5 days to appear.	→ Some foods may reduce the absorption of levothyroxine, hence a gap between eating and taking levothyroxine should be maintained

Insulin

Examples	Insulin is prescribed by brand name. Brand names have been omitted from this book. • Rapid-acting: insulin lispro, insulin aspart • Short-acting: soluble insulin • Intermediate: isophane insulin • Long-acting: insulin glargine, insulin determir	→ Onset within 5 minutes, duration 2–5 hours → Onset in 30–60 minutes, duration up to 9 hours → Onset in 1–2 hours, duration 11–24 hours → Onset in 1 hour, thereafter consistent activity for ≥24 hours
Mode of action	• Exogenous insulin mimics the action of endogenous insulin, a naturally occurring hormone that binds to the α subunit on the insulin receptor. This activates tyrosine kinase on ß subunit.	→ These cellular reactions result in the recruitment of glucose cell transporters to muscle and fat tissue, which increases glucose uptake by target tissues, increases glycogen synthesis in the liver, inhibits glycogenolysis and gluconeogenesis in the liver
Route of delivery	• S/C, IV (only in diabetic emergencies)	→ Insulin is inactivated by GI enzymes, hence it should be injected → Never abbreviate 'UNITS' in an insulin prescription
Indications	• Type 1 diabetes mellitus • Type 2 diabetes mellitus • Diabetic ketoacidosis and hyperglycaemic hyperosmolar non-ketotic coma (HONK) • Hyperkalaemia	→ 1st line drug for type 1 diabetics → Used when diet and other anti-diabetic agents have failed → Normally prescribed as a sliding scale regimen or as per protocol → Follow local hyperkalaemia guidelines
Cautions and contraindications	• Hypoglycaemia • Allergy to porcine or bovine insulins (note that some patients may have personal objections to taking insulins from these animals for religious or cultural reasons) • Insulin requirements may decrease in renal or hepatic impairment • Insulin requirements may change during pregnancy and breastfeeding	→ Monitor blood glucose before prescribing a dose of insulin → Human and analogue insulins exist as an alternative → Dose adjustment may be required → It is advisable that the patient's insulin doses are reviewed by an experienced diabetes physician during pregnancy or breastfeeding
Monitoring	• Monitor blood glucose and HbA1c as per local guidelines	→ To monitor glycaemic control
Interactions	• ACEi, beta blockers, corticosteroids, alcohol	→ Increased hypoglycaemic effect when used with insulin
Side-effects	• Common: – Hypoglycaemia – Lipoma at injection site (if injection sites not varied) – Local reactions at injection sites e.g. transient oedema	

| Patient counselling | • **Compliance and lifestyle measures:** explain the importance of compliance with treatment and instruct patients how to inject insulin safely and to dispose of sharps (single use insulin needles).
• **Insulin devices:** never extract insulin from a pen device as this can lead to fatal overdoses.
• **Provide verbal and written advice to patient regarding insulin use, hypoglycaemia and sick day rules:** inform patient of the risks and precautions with insulin use and provide written material.
• **Driving advice:** patients taking insulin or oral anti-diabetic drugs must inform the DVLA and their insurers about their diabetes. HGV drivers and drivers of public service vehicles must inform the DVLA about their diabetes, even if it is diet-controlled. | → Insulin should be injected into subcutaneous tissue in arms, thighs, abdomen and buttocks, and injection sites should be rotated

→ Patient information leaflets and Insulin Passports are widely available, along with online resources such as Diabetes UK (www.diabetes.org.uk) |

Insulin sick day rules (Diabetes UK):

How to manage insulin therapy during illness

- Stay well hydrated.
- Make contact with your diabetes team as soon as possible.
- Don't stop taking your insulin or other anti-diabetic medications even if you are eating less than normal (an exception to this is SGLT2 inhibitors which should not be taken by patients who are unwell and unable to eat). Dose adjustment may be required and advice can be sought from a diabetes team if you are unsure what to do.
- Test your blood sugar at least every four hours in illness.
- If your blood sugar is 15 mmol/L or more, check your urine for ketones. If ketones are present, contact your diabetes team.
- If your appetite is reduced or you are feeling nauseous and struggling to keep food down, replace meals with snacks or drinks containing carbohydrates, which will provide energy. Try to take sips of sugary drinks (such as fruit juice or non-diet cola or lemonade) or suck on glucose tablets or sweets such as jelly beans.
- If you are vomiting and unable to keep fluids down, seek medical help immediately.

Hypoglycaemia advice (Diabetes UK):

Preventing hypoglycaemia

- Don't miss a meal
- Eat enough carbohydrates for planned insulin intake
- Eat more carbohydrates if you are more active than normal
- Take your tablets or insulin injections as directed
- Do not drink alcohol on an empty stomach and do not drink excessive amounts of alcohol

Recognize signs of hypoglycaemia

A person who is having a hypoglycaemic episode ('hypo'), in which their blood sugar goes below 4 mmol/L, may develop the following symptoms: fatigue, hunger, sweating, shaking and pallor, blurred vision, lack of concentration, headaches and mood changes.

Treatment of hypoglycaemia and emergency kit

If you are conscious when having a hypo, you should consume 15–20 g of a fast-acting carbohydrate immediately e.g. glucose tablets or sweets such as jelly babies. Alternatively, drink some fruit juice or ordinary (non-diet) fizzy drink.

If you are unconscious when having a hypo and unable to swallow, another person will have to administer treatment to you. This will involve putting you in the recovery position and administering a glucagon injection (normally contained within a hypoglycaemia kit) if trained to give the injection. If a glucagon kit is not available or no one is trained to give the glucagon injection, an ambulance should be called immediately. If the patient does not recover within 10 minutes of treatment with glucagon, an ambulance should be called. Patients who are at risk of hypoglycaemia should carry with them at all times food for emergency treatment or a hypoglycaemia kit. It is also advisable that they should wear a medical alert bracelet or carry a diabetes card, and carry identification with them at all times.

Biguanides

Examples	• Metformin	
Mode of action	• Increase insulin sensitivity and reduce gluconeogenesis	→ Exact mechanism not fully understood
Route of delivery	• PO	→ Should be taken with food or after a meal
Indications	• Type 2 diabetes mellitus • Diabetes in pregnancy, both pre-existing diabetes and gestational diabetes • Polycystic ovarian syndrome (PCOS) – unlicensed use in the UK	→ 1st line drug for type 2 diabetes → Metformin should be discontinued after delivery in women with gestational diabetes → Women with PCOS tend to suffer from insulin resistance
Cautions and contraindications	• Acute kidney injury and severe renal impairment • Use with caution in lactic acidosis	→ Metformin can accumulate in these conditions → Withdraw metformin if patient develops lactic acidosis
Monitoring	• Monitor renal function before starting therapy and at least once a year	→ To establish and monitor baseline renal function for changes during therapy → If renal function deteriorates the patient may need dose adjustment or withdrawal of drug (if renal impairment severe enough)
Interactions	• Intravenous contrast media • ACEi, NSAIDs, diuretics • Prednisolone • Insulin and sulphonylureas	→ Metformin must be withheld 48 hours before and after a patient has had contrast media injected because both substances are nephrotoxic (large insult to the kidneys) → Interaction can cause AKI; monitor renal function → Elevates blood glucose, thus counteracting metformin → Increased possibility of hypoglycaemia
Side-effects	• Common: – Nausea and vomiting – Diarrhoea – Flatulence – Anorexia – Taste disturbance – Weight loss • Less common: – Lactic acidosis (rare) – Reduced vitamin B12 absorption (rare) • Frequency not known: – Hepatitis	• Mnemonic: **"Metformin is a biguanide, so you should give it to big people"** Metformin can promote weight loss so it may be useful in overweight or obese patients
Patient counselling	• **Treatment information:** • **Compliance and lifestyle measures:** • **Take with food:** • **Acidosis:** • **Driving advice:**	→ Explain to the patient why they should take metformin (indication and intended benefit) and the proposed duration of treatment. → Explain the importance of compliance with treatment and of lifestyle measures e.g. diet, exercise and smoking cessation. → Inform the patient that metformin should be taken with food or after a meal. → Tell patient to seek urgent medical attention if signs of acidosis occur, e.g. shallow breathing. → Patients taking insulin or oral anti-diabetic drugs must inform the DVLA and their insurers about their diabetes. HGV drivers and drivers of public service vehicles must inform the DVLA about their diabetes, even if it is diet-controlled.

Sulphonylureas

Examples	• Short-acting: gliclazide, tolbutamide	
	• Long-acting: glibenclamide, glimepiride	→ More likely to cause hypoglycaemia
Mode of action	• Stimulate insulin secretion from the pancreatic beta cells	→ If too much insulin is secreted by the beta cells, hypoglycaemia can occur
Routes of delivery	• PO	
Indications	• Type 2 diabetes mellitus	
Cautions and contraindications	• Ketoacidosis • Some sulphonylureas should be avoided in pregnancy and breastfeeding due to risk of hypoglycaemia in the infant • Use with caution in the elderly and in those with G6PD deficiency • Sulphonylureas may cause weight gain and therefore should only be prescribed in persistent poor diabetic control	
Interactions	• Insulin, other anti-diabetic drugs and alcohol	→ Increased risk of hypoglycaemia
	• ACEi and warfarin	→ These drugs possibly enhance the hypoglycaemic effect of sulphonylureas
Monitoring	• Monitoring of blood glucose and body weight during therapy	

Side-effects	• Less common:
	  – Hypoglycaemia
	  – GI upset
	  – Weight gain
	  – Blood disorders e.g. aplastic anaemia, agranulocytosis
	• Frequency not known:
	  – Hypersensitivity reactions
	  – Erythema multiforme
		• Mnemonic **WEIGHT GAIN HAPPENS (sulphonylurea side-effects)**
		Weight gain
		GI upset
		Hypoglycaemia

Patient counselling	• *Mode of action:*	→ Explain that this medication will help to reduce the patient's blood sugars by helping the body to produce more insulin. This medication will not cure the patient's diabetes and the patient will need to maintain a healthy diet and to exercise regularly.
	• *How to take:*	→ Sulphonylureas should be taken with food.
	• *Preventing hypoglycaemia:*	→ If prescribed in a patient who drives or operates machinery, warn the patient of the risk of hypoglycaemia and ask patient to consider their safety. Educate the patient about the signs of a hypoglycaemic attack and provide instructions about what the patient or people in the patient's surroundings should do in the event of a hypoglycaemic attack.

Patient counselling – **cont'd**	• **Weight gain:**	→ Warn patients that there is a risk of weight gain so it is important to monitor their weight.
	• **Surgery:**	→ Drug usually omitted on the morning of surgery.
	• **Driving advice:**	→ Patients taking insulin or oral anti-diabetic drugs must inform the DVLA and their insurers about their diabetes. HGV drivers and drivers of public service vehicles must inform the DVLA about their diabetes, even if it is diet-controlled.

Thiazolidinediones (glitazones)

Examples	• Pioglitazone, rosiglitazone	→ End in -glitazone
Mode of action	• Result in binding of the PPARγ-complex to DNA, which causes transcription of genes whose products are involved in insulin signalling (e.g. lipoprotein lipase, Glut-4) • Tissues also become more sensitive to insulin by recruiting glucose transporters to cell surfaces • This reduces peripheral insulin resistance, leading to a reduction of blood glucose concentration	→ Glitazones are only effective in the presence of insulin, so they can only be used in patients who have endogenous insulin production or who inject insulin
Route of delivery	• PO	
Indications	Used in type 2 diabetes mellitus in the following ways: • Single therapy: in overweight diabetic patients who cannot take metformin (contraindicated or not tolerated) • Dual therapy, with metformin or a sulphonylurea: when blood glucose control is not achieved with one drug and metformin and a sulphonyurea cannot be combined (contraindicated or not tolerated) • Triple therapy, with metformin and a sulphonylurea: when blood glucose control is inadequate (an alternative to starting insulin)	
Cautions and contraindications	• Avoid prescribing in patients with a history of heart failure • Avoid prescribing in previous or active bladder cancer and uninvestigated macroscopic haematuria • Avoid in pregnancy and breastfeeding, hepatic impairment and patients receiving dialysis • Use with caution in the elderly	→ There are concerns about increased incidence of heart failure in patients who take pioglitazone combined with insulin, particularly in those with cardiovascular risk factors; such patients require monitoring for signs of heart failure → There is a small increased risk of bladder cancer in patients who take pioglitazone → Increased risk of fractures
Monitoring	• Before starting pioglitazone treatment, assess patients for risk factors of bladder cancer and investigate any unexplained haematuria • Monitor closely for signs of heart failure especially in patients with a history of cardiovascular disease • Check LFTs at baseline and then every 2–6 months • Discontinue if patient develops jaundice	→ To reduce risk of bladder cancer
Interactions	• Insulin • Beta blockers • Other anti-diabetic drugs and alcohol	→ Increased risk of heart failure; use with caution → May mask signs of hypoglycaemia e.g. tremor → Increased risk of hypoglycaemia

Side-effects	• Common:
	  – Anaemia
	  – GI disturbances
	  – Weight gain
	  – Fluid retention
	  – Dizziness
	  – Headache
	  – Vertigo
	  – Visual disturbances
	  – Impotence
	  – Hypoaesthesia
	• Less common:
	  – Fatigue
	  – Alteration of blood lipids
	  – Hypoglycaemia
	  – Bladder cancer
	  – Liver dysfunction and liver toxicity
	  – Increased risk of bone fractures, especially in women	

Patient counselling	• ***Risks of treatment:*** • ***Alcohol:*** • ***Signs of liver toxicity:*** • ***Driving advice:***	→ Inform patient about side-effects and risks of treatment, including heart failure, bone fractures and bladder cancer. → It is not recommended to drink whilst on pioglitazone as this increases risk of hypoglycaemia. → The patient should be told to seek urgent medical help if they develop nausea, vomiting, abdominal pain, fatigue and dark urine. If the patient becomes jaundiced, they must stop taking the drug immediately and contact their doctor. → Patients taking insulin or oral anti-diabetic drugs must inform the DVLA and their insurers about their diabetes. HGV drivers and drivers of public service vehicles must inform the DVLA about their diabetes, even if it is diet-controlled.

DPP-4 inhibitors

Examples	• Sitagliptin, vidagliptin	➔ End in -gliptin
Mode of action	• Inhibit dipeptidylpeptidase-4, an enzyme which breaks down a type of gastrointestinal hormone called incretins	➔ Incretins increase insulin secretion and lower glucagon secretion
Routes of delivery	• PO	
Indications	• Type 2 diabetes which is resistant to 1st line treatment or add-on therapy	
Cautions and contraindications	• Contraindicated in pregnancy and breastfeeding • Avoid in diabetic ketoacidosis • Use with caution in renal insufficiency (may require dose adjustment), heart failure and in individuals with a history of pancreatitis	
Interactions	• Digoxin • Other anti-diabetic drugs and alcohol	➔ Increased plasma concentration of digoxin ➔ May increase risk of hypoglycaemia
Monitoring	• Baseline HbA1c and LFTs and check every 3 months	

Side-effects	• Common:
	  – GI disturbances
	  – Upper respiratory tract infections including nasopharyngitis
	  – Peripheral oedema
	  – Pain
	• Less common:
	  – Anorexia
	  – Pancreatitis
	  – Hepatotoxicity	

Patient counselling	• ***Beware of signs of liver impairment:*** • ***Beware of signs of pancreatitis:*** • ***Driving advice:***	➔ Seek medical help urgently if you notice pain in the right abdomen, nausea, vomiting or dark urine. ➔ Seek medical help immediately if you experience nausea, vomiting and severe abdominal pain. ➔ Patients taking insulin or oral anti-diabetic drugs must inform the DVLA and their insurers about their diabetes. HGV drivers and drivers of public service vehicles must inform the DVLA about their diabetes, even if it is diet-controlled.

Alpha-glucosidase inhibitors

Examples	• Acarbose	
Mode of action	• Delay the digestion and absorption of starch and sucrose, which lowers blood glucose levels	
Route of delivery	• PO	
Indications	• Type 2 diabetes mellitus, usually prescribed when other anti-glycaemic agents have failed, were contraindicated or not tolerated	
Cautions and contraindications	• Inflammatory bowel disease (IBD), hernia, previous abdominal surgery • Hepatic impairment • Pregnancy and breastfeeding	
Monitoring	• Monitor liver function by checking LFTs	
Interactions	• Digoxin • Alcohol • Orlistat (a drug that is a lipase inhibitor and is used as an adjunct in obesity)	→ Plasma concentration of digoxin reduced by acarbose → Increased risk of hypoglycaemia → Manufacturer advises against concomitant use of acarbose and orlistat

Side-effects	• Common:
	  – Abdominal pain
	  – Flatulence
	  – Diarrhoea and soft stools
	  – Abdominal distension
	• Less common:
	  – Abnormal LFTs, jaundice and hepatitis
	  – Skin reactions
	  – Oedema	

Patient counselling	• ***Carry glucose with you at all times:*** • ***Take with food:*** • ***Driving advice:***	→ Due to the risk of hypoglycaemia, especially if also taking insulin or sulphonylureas, patients should be advised to carry glucose (not sucrose) with them in the event of a hypoglycaemic episode. → Tablets should be swallowed whole immediately before meal or taken with first mouthful. → Patients taking insulin or oral anti-diabetic drugs must inform the DVLA and their insurers about their diabetes. HGV drivers and drivers of public service vehicles must inform the DVLA about their diabetes, even if it is diet-controlled.

Glucagon-like peptide-1 (GLP-1) receptor agonists

Examples	• Exenatide, liraglutide	→ End in -tide
Mode of action	• Bind to, and activate, the GLP-1 (glucagon-like peptide-1) receptor to increase insulin secretion, suppress glucagon secretion, and slow gastric emptying	
Routes of delivery	• S/C	
Indications	• Type 2 diabetes	
Cautions and contraindications	• Diabetic ketoacidosis • Severe GI disease • Pregnancy and breastfeeding • Use with caution in the elderly and in renal impairment	
Interactions	• Warfarin • Other anti-diabetic drugs, alcohol, steroids	→ Increased anticoagulant effect → Increased risk of hypoglycaemia
Monitoring	• Monitor the patient's HbA1c and blood glucose every 6 months • Monitor the patient's weight	

Side-effects	• Common:
	  – GI upset
	  – Weight loss
	• Less common:
	  – Severe pancreatitis
	  – Hypoglycaemia
	  – Anaphylactic reactions
		
		→ The pancreatitis can become haemorrhagic or necrotizing

Patient counselling	• ***Not with food:*** • ***Missed doses:*** • ***Concomitant use of medications:*** • ***When to seek help:*** • ***Stop immediately in acute pancreatitis:*** • ***Driving advice:*** • ***Contraception:***	→ Do not take after a meal. → If you have missed a dose, take the next dose as scheduled. → Some drugs, e.g. sulphonylureas, will require dose adjustment if used concomitantly. → Seek medical help immediately if nausea, vomiting or severe abdominal pain occurs. → If it is suspected that acute pancreatitis has developed as a result of this drug, the drug must be stopped immediately in addition to seeking medical help. → Patients taking insulin or oral anti-diabetic drugs must inform the DVLA and their insurers about their diabetes. HGV drivers and drivers of public service vehicles must inform the DVLA about their diabetes, even if it is diet-controlled. → Guidance from the BNF states that women of child-bearing age should use effective contraception during treatment with modified-release exenatide and for 12 weeks after discontinuation.

Combined oral contraceptive pill (COCP)

Examples	• COCPs are prescribed by brand name. Examples include Microgynon, Zoely, Qlaira and Levest.	➤ You should refer to your local prescribing guidelines to check which option is preferred.
Efficacy	Statistics from *Obstetrics & Gynaecology* 4th edition (Impey and Child, 2012): • Perfect use (using the contraceptive exactly as intended by the manufacturer): 1 in 1000 women will become pregnant within 1 year of using the COCP as only method of contraception • Typical use (the way the contraceptive is used by the average woman): 5 in 100 women will become pregnant within 1 year of using COCP as only method of contraception	➤ No protection against STIs
Mode of action	• Contains oestrogen and progestogen, which inhibit ovulation by negative feedback to suppress LH and FSH release	➤ In addition to preventing ovulation, the COCP thins the endometrium and thickens cervical mucus
Route of delivery	• PO	
Indications	• Contraception • Control of menstrual cycle (regularity) or symptoms e.g. menorrhagia, dysmenorrhoea and premenstrual symptoms • Acne and hirsutism	

Cautions and contraindications	• Contraindicated in the following:
	  – Current breast cancer
	  – Smoker >35 years
	  – Migraine with aura
	  – BMI >40
	  – History of VTE, cerebrovascular disease or CVA, hypertension or thrombophilia
	• Avoid up to 6 weeks postpartum
	• Use with caution in women with IBD
		➤ Affects breast milk volume
		➤ Reduced absorption of oral contraception

Monitoring	• BP and weight prior to starting treatment and at every 3–6 months review, before issuing a repeat prescription	➤ To ensure that healthy blood pressure and BMI are maintained and that the pill is still safe for patient to take
Interactions	• Warfarin • St John's wort, some antibiotics, antihypertensives and anti-epileptic drugs	➤ The pill reduces efficacy of warfarin ➤ May reduce contraceptive efficacy

Side-effects	• Common:
	  – Breast tenderness
	  – Breakthrough bleeding
	  – Headaches
	  – Nausea
	  – Cycle control
		• Mnemonic **COCP (COCP side-effects)**
		Cycle control
		Occasional irregular bleeding
		Clotting, **C**VD and **C**ancer (breast, cervical) more likely
		Pain (breast tenderness, headaches)

COCP – cont'd

Side-effects – **cont'd**	• Rare:
	  – Increased risk of VTE and CVD (MI, stroke)
	  – Increased risk of breast and cervical cancer

Patient counselling	• ***Efficacy:*** the COCP is not 100% efficacious in protection against unwanted pregnancies and does not protect against sexually transmitted diseases, so it is advisable to combine the COCP with a barrier method. This is a user-dependent method of contraception; hence it is the responsibility of the patient to remember to take the pill. If compliance is poor, the patient would be advised to consider a non-user dependent method or to use a barrier method.

Right column annotations (linked to corresponding bullets):

→ There are specific phone applications that can be downloaded to help women remember to take their pills on time.

• ***How to take the pill:*** normally start taking the pill on day 1 of cycle, take for 21 days and then have a pill-free week. However, the pill can be started at any day in the cycle provided extra precautions (e.g. use of a barrier method) are taken for 7 days.

→ Some brands contain 7 'dummy' pills that are taken instead of having the pill-free interval. These are placebo tablets that do not contain any hormones. Some women find it easier to take pills constantly than to have a break.

• ***Missed pills:*** if the patient misses the pill, she should take it as soon as she remembers (even if this means taking two pills together if more than 24 hours late). If the patient misses more than 2 pills, she is not protected against pregnancy and extra precautions should be taken for 7 days.

→ Strongly advise the patient to read the specific patient information leaflet for her pill regarding what to do in the event of missed pills, diarrhoea and vomiting. This leaflet is contained in the pill package and can be found online in many cases.

• ***Vomiting and diarrhoea:*** if the patient vomits within two hours of taking the pill, another pill should be taken. If severe vomiting and diarrhoea persist for more than 24 hours, additional precautions should be taken for 7 days.

• ***Antibiotics and the oral contraceptive pill:*** there have been some recent changes in guidelines regarding antibiotics and the use of the oral contraceptive pill. No additional contraceptive precautions are now required when combined oral contraceptives are used with antibiotics which do not induce liver enzymes, unless diarrhoea or vomiting occur.

→ Please review the BNF or the FSRH guidelines for more information.

• ***Adverse side-effects:*** inform patient about the side-effects of the COCP (including the increased risk of VTE, stroke and MI) and warn the patient to seek medical help immediately if she develops chest pain, leg pain and calf swelling, shortness of breath or haemoptysis.

• ***Emergency contraception and smoking cessation:*** offer advice regarding emergency contraception and smoking cessation.

→ It is preferred that a woman does not smoke when taking the COCP because it is an additional risk factor for cardiovascular and cerebrovascular events.

• ***Switching contraceptive:*** contact your GP or family planning clinic if you wish to switch to another contraceptive and they will advise you how to change your medication in a safe manner without compromising contraceptive cover.

• ***Surgery and the contraceptive pill:*** it may be necessary to stop the contraceptive pill for a period before or after having an operation due to the increased risk of VTE. However, it should be clarified with the surgical team undertaking the operation if this is necessary and the duration.

Combined vaginal ring

Examples	• Combined vaginal rings are prescribed by brand name.	→ At present only NuvaRing is licensed for use in the UK, but refer to your local prescribing guidelines to check if an alternative option is preferred.
Efficacy	• Similar efficacy to COCP (see p. 57)	→ No protection against STIs
Mode of action	• Contains oestrogen and progestogen, which inhibit ovulation by negative feedback to suppress LH and FSH release • Thins endometrium and thickens cervical mucus	
Routes of delivery	• Ring pessary	→ Latex-free ring which the patient inserts into the vagina and leaves in place for 3 weeks → Applicator available to ease insertion
Indications	• Contraception • Control of menstrual cycle (regularity) or symptoms e.g. menorrhagia, dysmenorrhoea and premenstrual symptoms	

Cautions and contraindications	• Same as for COCP, with the following exceptions:
	  – Women with IBD will not have absorption problems as the ring has a local effect
	  – Women with vaginal prolapse may struggle to keep the ring in place	

Interactions	• Same as COCP (see p. 57)	
Monitoring	• Same as COCP (see p. 57)	

Side-effects	• Common:
	  – Headache
	  – Discomfort
	  – Vaginal discharge
	  – Irregular bleeding (less likely than with COCP)
	• Rare:
	  – Increased risk of VTE, CVD (MI, stroke), breast and cervical cancer	

Patient counselling	• **Side-effects:** explain the side-effects of the vaginal ring. • **Insertion:** ensure that the patient understands how to insert ring and offer to demonstrate insertion if she is uncertain.	→ It is preferred that the patient inserts the vaginal ring on day 2–5 of her cycle. However, the ring can be inserted at any time during the cycle as long as extra precautions (e.g. a condom) are used for 7 days.

Combined vaginal ring – *cont'd*

| Patient counselling – **cont'd** | • **How to take:** explain that the patient should insert the ring into the vagina and keep it in for 3 weeks and then remove it for one week to have a withdrawal bleed. The ring can be taken out of the vagina for up to 3 hours, without compromising contraceptive cover.
• **Missed doses:** if the patient forgets to remove a ring after 3 weeks or to insert a ring after the one-week break, extra precautions are needed for 7 days.
• **Daily use:** the ring can be worn during all activities, including intercourse, but there is a risk that the ring could fall out or that the ring could break. It is possible that the patient will be aware of the ring's presence and that a partner might feel it during sex. | → There are special instructions for what to do if the ring falls out or breaks, with regard to washing and replacement. Strongly advise patient to read information leaflet provided with vaginal ring. |

Combined transdermal patch

Examples	• Transdermal patches are prescribed by brand name.	→ At present only the Evra patch is licensed for use in the UK, but refer to your local prescribing guidelines to check if an alternative option is preferred.
Efficacy	• Similar efficacy to other combined hormonal contraception; no protection against STIs	
Mode of action	• Releases oestrogen and progestogen transdermally, which thin endometrium and thicken cervical mucus	→ These endometrial and cervical changes reduce the chance of fertilization by sperm and implantation of an egg
Routes of delivery	• Topical (patch)	
Indications	• Same as combined vaginal ring (see p. 59)	
Cautions and contraindications	• Same as COCP (see p. 57), with the addition: – Women over 90 kg	→ The contraceptive patch is not as effective in this group
Interactions	• Same as COCP, with the exception of warfarin	
Monitoring	• BP and weight should be monitored during therapy	
Side-effects	• Same as COCP (see p. 57)	
Patient counselling	• *Side-effects:* the side-effects of combined hormonal contraception and local skin irritation can occur. • *How to use:* explain that the patch should be applied topically and kept in place for 3 weeks, then removed for 1 week and a new patch applied. If the patch is off for more than 48 consecutive hours during the 3 weeks, contraceptive cover is compromised. Advise patient to read information leaflet for full instructions.	• Mnemonic **PATCH (combined transdermal patch side-effects)** **P**ain (breast tenderness, headaches) **A**menorrhoea **T**endency to put on weight (increased appetite) **C**lots and cancer more likely (breast, cervical) **H**ypertension (BP may rise)

Progestogen-only pill (POP)

Examples	• POPs are prescribed by brand name.	→ Examples of POPs include Noriday (traditional) and Cerazette (desogestrel-based). Refer to your local prescribing guidelines to see which is preferred.
Efficacy	Statistics from *Obstetrics & Gynaecology* 4th edition (Impey and Child, 2012): • Perfect use (using the contraceptive exactly as intended by the manufacturer): 5 in 1000 women will become pregnant within 1 year of using the POP as only method of contraception • Typical use (the way the contraceptive is used by the average woman): 5 in 100 women will become pregnant within 1 year of using POP as only method of contraception	→ No protection against STIs
Mode of action	• Contains progestogen, which causes thinning of the endometrium and thickens cervical mucus and inhibits ovulation in some women	→ Prevents fertilization of sperm and prevents implantation of a fertilized egg (should fertilization occur)
Routes of delivery	• PO	
Indications	• Contraception, usually offered to women who cannot take combined hormonal contraception • Control of menstrual cycle and symptoms, particularly women who wish to avoid periods	
Cautions and contraindications	• History of liver tumours • Genital and breast cancer • Undiagnosed vaginal bleeding • Severe arterial disease • Acute porphyria • Avoid in hepatic impairment	
Monitoring	• BP and weight should be monitored during therapy • Close monitoring of blood glucose for diabetic patients	→ POP reduces glucose metabolism and can worsen diabetic control
Interactions	• Anti-epileptic drugs, St John's wort	→ Reduced contraceptive effect

Side-effects	• Side-effects similar to COCP:
	  – Pain (breast tenderness and headaches)
	  – Increased appetite
	  – Irregular bleeding such as spotting (usually at the start of treatment; many women become amenorrhoeic on the POP)
	  – Mood changes
	• Side-effects different from COCP:
	  – Does not cause VTE
		• Mnemonic **POPs (progestogen-only pill side-effects)**
		Pain (breast tenderness, headaches)
		Overemotional (mood changes, premenstrual tension)
		Putting on weight (increased appetite)
		Spotting or **S**top of periods (amenorrhoea)

Patient counselling	• **Side-effects and protection against STIs:**	→	Explain side-effects of progestogen-only contraception and warn the patient that she may experience erratic bleeding, spotting or amenorrhoea. Remind the patient that the POP offers no protection against STIs.
	• **How to take:**	→	The POP is taken once daily and must be taken at the same time every day. If more than 3 hours have passed, contraceptive cover is compromised and extra precautions should be used. There are no breaks when taking the POP.
	• **Missed pill advice:**	→	There are two types of POPs, traditional POPs and desogestrel-containing POPs. If a traditional POP is less than 3 hours late or a desogestrel POP is less than 12 hours late, then the missed pill should be taken as soon as remembered. If more than one pill has been missed, only one pill should be taken. The next pill should be taken at the usual time. This may mean that two pills are taken in one day. Additional contraceptive precautions (condoms or avoidance of sex) are advised for 48 hours after restarting the POP. Emergency contraception is indicated if unprotected sexual intercourse occurred after the missed pill and within 48 hours of restarting the POP (Faculty of Sexual and Reproductive Health March 2015, Progestogen-only pills guidance). If the missed pills occur in other circumstances, the woman should contact her GP or family planning or sexual health services for more specific advice.

Contraceptive implants

Examples	• Contraceptive implants are prescribed by brand name.	→ At present only Nexplanon is licensed for use in the UK, but refer to your local prescribing guidelines to check if an alternative option is preferred.
Efficacy	Statistics from *Obstetrics & Gynaecology* 4th edition (Impey and Child, 2012): • 5 in 1000 women will become pregnant in 1 year • Non-user dependent method	→ No protection against STIs
Mode of action	• Subdermal release of progestogen, which thins the endometrium and thickens cervical mucus	→ The role of progestogen is to create an unfavourable environment for fertilization and implantation of an egg
Routes of delivery	• 40 mm rod inserted subdermally into the upper arm under local anaesthetic	
Indications	• Long-term reversible contraception which lasts up to 3 years	→ Take care not to confuse the contraceptive implant with the contraceptive injection, which also contains progestogen, but only lasts for 3 months and is not suitable for long-term use
Cautions and contraindications	• Same as POP (see p. 62)	
Interactions	• Same as POP (see p. 62)	
Monitoring	• Same as POP (see p. 62)	
Side-effects	• In addition to the progestogenic side-effects, the patient might experience: – Skin irritation at site of insertion	
Patient counselling	• ***Side-effects and duration of action:*** explain the side-effects of the contraceptive implant and that it is active for 3 years, after which it will need replacing. • ***Trial of POPs first:*** depending on local practice – the following is advised by some family planning clinics – the patient may need to have a trial of POPs to see how her body reacts to progestogen before having the procedure. If this is the case, please explain the rationale behind this trial of progestogen. • ***No risk of losing implant in arm:*** reassure patient that the contraceptive implant can be detected by X-rays and will not be 'lost' in the arm. This has been a concern for women in the past and the implants inserted these days are made of a radio-opaque material.	→ The most common cause of a request for early removal of the implant is erratic bleeding. To reduce the likelihood of inconvenience to the patient resulting in early removal, the patient is sometimes given a trial of progestogen-only pills. If she does not experience erratic bleeding during this trial or the bleeding resolves, a decision is made to insert the contraceptive implant.

Intrauterine system (IUS)

Examples	• Intrauterine systems are prescribed by name.	➤ At present only three are licensed for use in the UK – Mirena, Levosert and Jaydess. You should refer to your local prescribing guidelines to check which option is preferred.
Efficacy	Statistics from *Obstetrics & Gynaecology* 4th edition (Impey and Child, 2012): • 2 in 1000 women will become pregnant within 1 year • Non-user dependent method	➤ No protection against STIs
Mode of action	• Releases progestogen locally, which thins the endometrium, thickens cervical mucus and suppresses ovulation in some women	
Routes of delivery	• Plastic device which sits in uterus	➤ Intrauterine release of hormones
Indications	• Contraception • Menorrhagia • Protection from endometrial hyperplasia during oestrogen replacement therapy	➤ Reduces menstrual flow
Cautions and contraindications	• Same as POP (see p. 62)	
Interactions	• Same as POP (see p. 62)	
Monitoring	• Same as POP (see p. 62)	

Side-effects	• The progestogen released by the IUS is local and low in concentration so many of the systemic side-effects of progestogen occur less often than with the POP (see p. 62)
	• Specific risks of IUS:
	  – Infection
	  – Expulsion
	  – Perforation
	  – Ectopic pregnancy
		• Mnemonic **Progestogenic IUS (IUS risks)**
		Progestogenic (local) side-effects
		Infection & **I**ncorrectly placed pregnancy (ectopic)
		Unintentional puncture (perforation)
		Slipping out (expulsion)

Patient counselling	• *Risks and benefits:* • *Side-effects and duration of action:*	➤ Explain the side-effects of progestogen-only contraception and specific risks of IUS. ➤ Explain that the IUS is active for 3–5 years (depending on brand), after which it will need replacing. Inform patient that she may have irregular bleeding in the first 6 months of IUS insertion; however, she should experience lighter bleeds and may even become amenorrhoeic.

IUS – *cont'd*

Patient counselling – **cont'd**	• ***When to seek medical help:***	Warn the patient to seek medical help immediately if she experiences severe abdominal pain or severe vaginal bleeding.
	• ***Perforation and ectopic pregnancy:***	Warn patient about the risks of perforation and inform her that if she were to get pregnant whilst on the IUS, her pregnancy is more likely to be an ectopic pregnancy (i.e. pregnancy outside the womb), although this is a rare complication.
	• ***Expulsion and checking threads:***	Warn patient that expulsion can occur and this is most likely to occur within weeks of insertion. The IUS has threads that the patient can feel to ensure the IUS is in place.

Intrauterine contraceptive devices (IUCD, also known as the copper coil)

Examples	• Intrauterine devices are prescribed by name. Examples include Ancora, GyneFix, Multi-Safe and Novaplus.	➤ You should refer to your local prescribing guidelines to check which option is preferred.
Efficacy	Statistics from *Obstetrics & Gynaecology* 4th edition (Impey and Child, 2012): • 1 in 100 will get pregnant in one year • Non-user dependent method	➤ No protection against STIs
Mode of action	• Does not contain any hormones, but acts as a physical barrier to fertilization and is spermicidal	
Routes of delivery	• Intrauterine spermicidal barrier to fertilization	
Indications	• Long-term reversible contraception • Emergency contraception	➤ Can be inserted within 5 days of unprotected intercourse
Cautions and contraindications	• Caution in menorrhagia and dysmenorrhoea as the IUCD often causes periods to become heavier and more painful	
Interactions	• None	
Monitoring	• None, unless patient seeks medical help	

Side-effects	• Common:
	  – Heavier and more painful periods
	  – Risk of infection
	• Less common:
	  – Expulsion
	  – Perforation
	  – Ectopic pregnancy
		• Mnemonic **IUCD (IUCD risks)**
		Infection and **I**ncorrectly placed pregnancy (ectopic)
		Unintentional puncture (perforation)
		Crampy heavy period
		Drop (expulsion)

Patient counselling	• *Risks*: • *Duration of 5 years:*	➤ Explain the risks of IUCDs, including ectopic pregnancy, perforation and expulsion. Warn patient to seek medical help immediately if she experiences severe abdominal pain or severe vaginal bleeding. ➤ Explain that the copper coil is active for 5 years before needing replacement.

Prescribing in pregnancy:

Physiological changes in pregnancy and teratogenicity:

- There are a number of physiological changes that occur in pregnancy that change how drugs are absorbed and metabolized by the pregnant woman.
- Some drugs may have an adverse impact on the growing fetus.
- A drug that is harmful to a growing fetus or an unborn child is known as a teratogen.
- It is important for a prescriber to have knowledge about teratogens and to stop them before they cause harm.

Timing and exposure to teratogens:

- The 1st trimester, i.e. the first three months of pregnancy, is the time during the pregnancy in which the risk of congenital abnormalities occurring is the greatest.
- The 2nd and 3rd trimesters pose risks due to toxicity to fetal tissues with exposure to teratogens.
- After childbirth there are drugs that can be passed to an infant through breastfeeding and they may cause harm. Therefore, mothers should check manufacturers' leaflets for the medications they are taking to ensure that they are safe to take during lactation.

Dangerous medications in pregnancy:

- Known teratogens include warfarin (p. 11), anti-epileptic medications (p. 88), some anti-hypertensive drugs such as ACEi (p. 2) and ARBs (p. 4), some antibiotics e.g. trimethoprim (p. 118) and tetracycline (p. 113), cytotoxic agents (p. 94) and lithium (p. 81). See relevant pages for more information on individual drug teratogenicity.

Advice for prescribing in pregnancy:

- Avoid starting new medications during the first trimester.
- Only prescribe a medication if absolutely necessary and use the lowest effective dose.
- Try to establish symptomatic control over chronic medical conditions that require drug therapy, e.g. diabetes and hypothyroidism, prior to conception.
- Avoid making medication changes during pregnancy.
- Advise pregnant women to take folic acid during their pregnancy to reduce the risk of neural tube defects.
- Since many pregnancies are unplanned, NICE guidelines recommend that healthcare professionals should advise all women who may become pregnant to take folic acid (NICE 2008, PH11).
- Avoid prescribing teratogenic drugs in women of child-bearing age as they could become pregnant unintentionally. If it is essential to prescribe a teratogenic drug to manage a condition, ensure that the patient is using appropriate contraception and that she is aware of the teratogenic risks of the drug.
- If a woman is confirmed to be pregnant, it is essential to stop any teratogenic drugs.
- Advise pregnant women to abstain from smoking because of the risk of complications such as intrauterine growth restriction and increased risk of ectopic pregnancy.
- Advise pregnant women to maintain a healthy diet and get adequate sleep and rest to cope better with the physical demands of pregnancy.

Phosphodiesterase type 5 (PDE5) inhibitors

Examples	• Sildenafil, vardenafil, tadalafil	→ End in -afil
Mode of action	• Inhibit phosphodiesterase type 5 (PDE5), which is found in the corpus cavernosum of the penis and in the lungs and breaks down cyclic guanosine monophosphate (cGMP) • cGMP is found naturally in the lungs but is produced following sexual stimulation (triggered by NO release)	→ cGMP causes relaxation and vasodilatation of the peripheral arteries, and increased blood flow to the penis results in penile engorgement → Inhibition of cGMP breakdown will increase cGMP levels and this will relieve pulmonary hypertension and improve the ability of a male to have an erection
Routes of delivery	• PO, IV	
Indications	• Erectile dysfunction • Pulmonary arterial hypertension	
Cautions and contraindications	• Hypotension • Recent stroke or myocardial infarction • Unstable angina • Concurrent use of nitrates • Patients with hereditary retinal disorders e.g. retinitis pigmentosa • Use with caution in cardiovascular disease, left ventricular outflow obstruction and in patients who are prone to priapism or have anatomical deformities of the penis	→ Do not prescribe if the patient's systolic BP <90 mmHg → Risk of severe hypotension → Phosphodiesterase type 5 inhibitors may act on phosphodiesterase type 6, which is found in the retina and is important to the maintenance of vision
Interactions	• Nitrates, nicorandil, alpha blockers, CCBs • Other PDE5 inhibitors • Grapefruit juice	→ Severe hypotension can occur due to vasodilatation → Use of more than one PDE5 inhibitor is not recommended → May increase plasma concentrations of sildenafil
Monitoring	• Ask patient about drug efficacy and adverse effects	

Side-effects	• Common:
	  – Back pain
	  – Migraine
	  – Flushing
	  – Hypotension
	  – Visual disturbance
	  – Nasal congestion
	• Rare:
	  – Priapism
	  – Non-arteritic anterior ischaemic optic neuropathy
	  – Sudden vision loss
		→ Some of these side-effects, such as flushing, migraine and hypotension, are caused by vasodilatation of other vascular beds

PDE5 inhibitors – *cont'd*

Patient counselling	• *How to take medication:*	If taken orally for erectile dysfunction, tablets should be taken an hour before intercourse; the onset of effect can be delayed if the tablets are taken with food.
	• *When to seek help:*	The patient should seek medical help if the erection is maintained for longer than 2 hours.
	• *Visual changes:*	Tell the patient to report visual changes to their doctor as soon as they arise.

5α-reductase inhibitors

Examples	• Finasteride, dutasteride	→ End in -steride
Mode of action	• Inhibit 5α-reductase, an enzyme that metabolizes testosterone into dihydrotestosterone (more potent)	→ This results in a reduction in prostate size, which improves urinary and obstructive symptoms
Route of delivery	• PO	
Indications	• Benign prostatic hypertrophy • Male pattern baldness (finasteride)	
Cautions and contraindications	• Women who are pregnant or of child-bearing age and sexually active must avoid exposure to 5α-reductase inhibitors. They should not handle broken tablets or leaking capsules of finasteride and if they are having intercourse with a man who takes 5α-reductase inhibitors, a condom should be used as such drugs are excreted in the semen. • Use with caution in obstructive uropathy	→ Teratogenic: cause abnormal development of external genitalia in a male fetus
Monitoring	• Review treatment at 3–6 months and then every 6–12 months	→ Caution if checking PSA, as PSA values are affected by 5α-reductase inhibitor (different reference values used)
Interactions	• None	

Side-effects	• Less common:
	  – Breast cancer in male patients
	• Frequency not known:
	  – Loss of libido, impotence and gynaecomastia
	  – Suicidal ideation has been reported in men taking finasteride (MHRA/CHM guidance, May 2017)	

Patient counselling	• ***Mode of action and side-effects:*** • ***Women of child-bearing age should never be exposed to drug:*** • ***Report breast changes:***	→ Explain how the medication works and the side-effects, including reduced libido, impotence and gynaecomastia. → Inform the patient that it is very dangerous for a woman who is or could become pregnant to be exposed to a 5α-reductase inhibitor. These drugs should not be touched or handled by such women. If the patient has sex with a woman of child-bearing age, he should wear a condom. → Warn patient to tell their GP about changes in the breast tissue or discharge.

Alpha-adrenoceptor blockers (also known as alpha-adrenoceptor antagonists)		
Examples	• Tamsulosin, doxazosin, prazosin	→ End in -osin
Mode of action	• Inhibit alpha adrenoceptors to relax smooth muscle in blood vessels and in the urinary tract	→ This improves circulation and reduces resistance in the blood vessels (which in turn lowers blood pressure) → When the muscles in the urinary tract are relaxed, it is easier to pass urine
Routes of delivery	• PO	
Indications	• Benign prostatic hypertrophy (tamsulosin) • Hypertension (doxazosin, prazosin)	
Cautions and contraindications	• Avoid in patients with a history of postural hypotension or micturition syncope • Use with caution in patients undergoing cataract surgery • Use with caution in elderly patients	→ Risk of intraoperative floppy iris syndrome → Increased risk of postural hypotension
Interactions	• Anti-hypertensive drugs, MAOIs and PDE5 inhibitors • Digoxin • NSAIDs • Ketoconazole	→ Increased risk of severe hypotension → Prazosin increases plasma concentration of digoxin → NSAIDs antagonize hypotensive effect of alpha-adrenoceptor blockers → Ketoconazole increases plasma concentration of tamsulosin
Monitoring	• Review patient 4–6 weeks into treatment and enquire about urinary symptoms (if treated for BPH) • Check lying and standing BP (if treated for HTN)	

Side-effects	• Frequency not known:
	  – Postural hypotension
	  – Blurred vision
	  – Dry mouth
	  – Dizziness
	  – Drowsiness
	  – Syncope
	  – Gastrointestinal disturbances
	  – Hypersensitivity reactions
	  – Oedema
	  – Intraoperative floppy iris syndrome (tamsulosin and doxazosin)
	  – Erectile disorders (such as retrograde ejaculation)	

Patient counselling	• **Postural hypotension:**	→ Warn the patient about postural hypotension and suggest that the drug is taken at night.
	• **Impaired driving:**	→ Warn patients on doxazosin or tamsulosin that these drugs may cause drowsiness which can impair a patient's ability to drive.
	• **Can take time to work:**	→ If prescribed for BPH, inform patient that it can take a couple of weeks to notice a significant improvement in urinary symptoms.
	• **Lifestyle measures:**	→ If prescribed for treatment of hypertension, counsel patient on lifestyle measures such as weight loss and smoking cessation.
	• **Unwanted side-effect:**	→ Male patients should be informed that tamsulosin can cause erectile disorders such as retrograde ejaculation. This is a side-effect that can cause distress to some men.

Selective serotonin reuptake inhibitors (SSRIs)

Examples	• Citalopram, fluoxetine, paroxetine, sertraline	
Mode of action	• Selectively inhibit serotonin reuptake in the synaptic cleft, so that the amount of serotonin in the brain is increased to normal levels	➤ Serotonin is a neurotransmitter which is strongly involved in mood regulation ➤ Depression has been linked to low serotonin levels
Routes of delivery	• PO	
Indications	• Depression • Generalized anxiety disorder • Depressive illness in children (fluoxetine only) • Panic disorder (citalopram) • Obsessive–compulsive disorder (sertraline) • Bulimia nervosa (fluoxetine)	➤ 1st line in depression ➤ Sertraline has the strongest evidence base for treating depression in patients who are post-MI ➤ Note that fluoxetine is associated with an increased risk of self-harm and suicidal ideation, which needs to be monitored
Cautions and contraindications	• Contraindicated in pregnancy, in poorly controlled epilepsy and during manic phases • Use with caution in patients with epilepsy, cardiac disease, diabetes or receiving electroconvulsive therapy (ECT) • Use with caution in patients who are prone to acute angle-closure glaucoma or have a history of bleeding disorders	
Interactions	• Alcohol • NSAIDs and aspirin • Anti-epileptic drugs • Theophylline • Monoamine oxidase inhibitors (MAOIs) • Tramadol and St John's wort • Grapefruit interacts with sertraline via CYP3A4 inhibition	➤ Increased sedation ➤ Increased risk of bleeding; consider co-prescribing a gastro-protective drug in older people taking NSAIDs or aspirin with an SSRI (NICE 2009, CG90) ➤ Reduced seizure threshold ➤ SSRI potentiates effect of theophylline, so halve the dose or avoid theophylline ➤ MAOIs should not be started until at least a week after an SSRI has been stopped (5 weeks in the case of fluoxetine). Conversely, SSRIs should not be started until 2 weeks after stopping an MAOI (BNF 2017) ➤ Increased risk of serotonin discontinuation syndrome ➤ Increased plasma concentration of sertraline *Please note that grapefruit interactions are drug-specific, not class-specific*

Monitoring	• Review patient every 1–2 weeks initially after starting an SSRI. Consider switching antidepressant if the patient does not respond after at least 1 month of treatment (or if the patient does not respond in 6 weeks in the case of elderly patients). Continue drug for an additional 2–4 weeks in cases of partial response (BNF 2017) • Following remission, antidepressant treatment should be continued at the same dose for at least 6 months (about 12 months in the elderly), or for at least 12 months in patients receiving treatment for generalized anxiety disorder (as the likelihood of relapse is high). Patients with a history of recurrent depression should receive maintenance treatment for at least 2 years (BNF 2017) • Follow-up should be arranged for patients after cessation of treatment with an antidepressant	→ Ask the patient about suicidal ideation and self-harm
Side-effects	• Common: – GI upset – Nausea – Hyponatraemia – Dry mouth – Sexual dysfunction – Anorexia and weight loss • Less common: – Increased risk of bleeding – Suicidal ideation – Convulsions – QT interval prolongation – Serotonin syndrome – SSRI discontinuation syndrome	• Mnemonic **SSRIs (SSRI side-effects)** **S**ore tummy (GI upset) **S**exual dysfunction **R**educed weight and reduced salivation (dry mouth) **I**ncreased risk of bleeding and convulsions **S**erotonin toxicity and **S**erotonin discontinuation syndrome → Consider co-prescribing gastro-protective agent → Syndrome resulting from increased serotonin activity → Occurs most frequently after cessation of paroxetine therapy, as it is the SSRI with the shortest $t_{1/2}$
Patient counselling	• *Mode of action and side-effects:* • *Lifestyle measures:* • *Onset of effect and compliance:*	→ Inform the patient about how the SSRI works and about the possible side-effects, which tend to be mild and transient. → Explain the importance of regular exercise, maintaining a healthy diet and getting adequate sleep, as these factors may improve the patient's mood. Cognitive behavioural therapy and counselling may also help but sometimes these services can have long waiting lists. → Explain that SSRIs can take a couple of weeks to start working and the first sign that the patient may notice is better sleep. It is important to persist with treatment in the first few weeks even if the patient feels like the SSRI is not working.

SSRIs – *cont'd*		
Patient counselling – **cont'd**	• *Duration of treatment:*	→ Inform the patient that they will have to continue taking the antidepressant for a period after their depressive symptoms have improved and that the amount of time will depend on the severity of their depression. The patient must be informed that there is a risk of relapse and that if relapse occurs the patient should contact their doctor for further management.
	• *Withdrawal:*	→ If the patient wishes to come off the antidepressant, the withdrawal will have to occur gradually.
	• *Switching antidepressants:*	→ If they are being switched from one antidepressant to another, they might need to come off the first antidepressant completely and take a short break before restarting the second antidepressant, to avoid dangerous drug interactions.
	• *Serotonin syndrome:*	→ Counsel the patient about the signs of serotonin syndrome (agitation, confusion, nystagmus, myoclonus, tremor, seizures, hyperpyrexia and autonomic instability). Advise them to seek medical help immediately if they suspect serotonin syndrome. Treatment includes stopping the drug and symptomatic management.
	• *Signs of SSRI discontinuation syndrome:*	→ Warn patients about the signs of SSRI discontinuation syndrome such as headache, paraesthesia, shock-like sensations, gastrointestinal symptoms, lethargy, insomnia and change in mood.

Tricyclic antidepressants (TCAs)

Examples	• Amitriptyline, nortriptyline, lofepramine, dosulepin, trazodone	
Mode of action	• Mechanism of action in depressive illness not fully understood, but believed to involve adaptive responses to monoaminergic neurotransmission	
Routes of delivery	• PO	
Indications	• Depression • Panic attacks and anxiety disorders • Neuralgia (e.g. amitriptyline) • Nocturnal enuresis	→ Unlicensed use
Cautions and contraindications	• Suicidal ideation • History of psychosis or bipolar disorder • QT interval prolongation • Avoid in patients post-MI or with other heart problems (consider sertraline in such patients) • Use with caution in prostatic hypertrophy, urinary retention, chronic constipation, increased intraocular pressure, mania, severe liver disease and in those with a high risk of developing acute angle-closure glaucoma	→ TCAs more toxic in overdose compared to alternatives → TCAs may aggravate these conditions and should be avoided
Interactions	• Monoamine oxidase inhibitors • Anti-epileptic medications • Anti-arrhythmic medications • Alcohol	→ Severe hypertensive crisis can occur; maintain a 2-week gap between stopping a TCA and starting an MAOI, and vice versa → TCAs lower the seizure threshold in epileptic patients → Ventricular tachycardia can occur → Increased sedation
Monitoring	• See SSRIs, as monitoring is similar	

Side-effects	• Elderly patients are more susceptible to all TCA side-effects, particularly hyponatraemia
	• Common:
	  – Antimuscarinic effects (dry mouth, blurred vision, constipation, urinary retention)
	  – Central nervous system effects (anxiety, restlessness, dizziness, agitation, confusion)
	  – Metabolic effects (weight gain, altered blood glucose in diabetics)
	• Less common:
	  – Cardiotoxic in overdose
	  – Neuroleptic malignant syndrome
	  – Hyponatraemia
		• Mnemonic **TCAs (TCA side-effects)**
		Thrombocytopenia
		Cardiac events (stroke, MI)
		Anticholinergic side-effects
		Seizures
		
		→ One of the reasons TCAs are not prescribed 1st line

TCAs – cont'd

Patient counselling		
	• *Impairment of normal abilities:*	→ Warn the patient that the TCA can cause drowsiness that may impair their ability to drive or operate machinery. If the patient drinks alcohol, they should be informed that they may experience increased sedation if consuming alcohol whilst on a TCA.
	• *Important not to exceed maximum dose:*	→ Explain to the patient that the drug is very dangerous in overdose. Prior to prescribing this drug, ascertain that the patient is not considering suicide or engaging in self-harming behaviours as this would put them at increased risk of intentionally overdosing.
	• *Increased risk of seizures in epilepsy:*	→ Warn patients who are epileptic that they may experience more seizures as this drug lowers the seizure threshold, making it easier for a seizure to occur, as a lower level of stimuli is required.
	• *Treatment cessation:*	→ Warn the patient that withdrawal symptoms may occur within 4 days of stopping drug. However, such symptoms tend to be mild and self-limiting. Drug should be withdrawn gradually over at least 4 weeks and this would depend on how long the patient has been taking the antidepressant and how they respond to withdrawal.

Monoamine oxidase inhibitors (MAOIs): *not prescribed as commonly as other types of antidepressants due to severe food and drug interactions*

Examples	• Reversible: moclobemide • Irreversible: phenelzine, isocarboxazid, tranylcypromine	➤ Thought to cause fewer food and drug interactions than irreversible MAOIs
Mode of action	• Inhibit monoamine oxidase, resulting in an increase in amine neurotransmitters	
Route of delivery	• PO	
Indications	• Depression which is refractory to treatment	➤ Works well in patients with phobia, or atypical hypochondriacal or hysterical features
Cautions and contraindications	• Contraindicated in cerebrovascular disease, phaeochromocytoma and in manic phases • Avoid concomitant use of other antidepressants • Avoid in pregnancy • Avoid in agitated patients • Use with caution in the elderly population and in patients who experience severe hypertensive reactions to certain drugs and foods • Use with caution in acute porphyria, cardiovascular disease, diabetes mellitus, concurrent ECT and surgery	➤ Severe CNS toxicity can occur ➤ Increased risk of neonatal malformations
Monitoring	• Ask about symptomatic improvement • Check blood pressure	➤ Drug may cause postural hypotension or hypertension
Interactions	• Food and drinks with a high tyramine content: mature cheese, hydrolysed meats or yeast extracts, wines, beers or other alcoholic drinks (including drinks with low alcohol), pickled foods, banana skins, broad bean pods • Other antidepressants • Carbamazepine	• Mnemonic **CHEAP (foods that interact with MAOIs)** **C**heese **H**ydrolysed meats **E**xtracts (yeast) **A**lcohol (wines, beers, low-alcohol drinks) **P**ickles, broad bean pods and banana skins

Side-effects	• Common or very common:
	  – Dizziness
	  – Postural hypotension
	• Uncommon:
	  – Behavioural changes including agitation
	  – Blurred vision
	  – Convulsions
	  – GI disturbances
	  – Deranged LFTs	

MAOIs – *cont'd*		
Side-effects – **cont'd**	• Rare: – Progressive hepatocellular necrosis that can be fatal • Note that hypertensive reaction with foods high in tyramine can occur • Withdrawal symptoms may occur on cessation (and such symptoms range in severity and nature)	→ Dangerous but less likely to occur with reversible MAOIs → Paranoid hallucinations and delusions can occur
Patient counselling	• ***Dangerous reaction to food and drinks:*** foods with high tyramine content such as mature cheeses, hydrolysed meats, pickled foods and alcohol interact with MAOIs. The BNF states that 'patients should be advised to eat only fresh foods and avoid food that is suspected of being stale or "going off". This is especially important with meat, fish, poultry or offal; game should be avoided. The danger of interaction persists for up to 2 weeks after treatment with MAOIs is discontinued'. (BNF 2017) • ***Do not take other antidepressants at the same time:*** explain the dangers of concomitant use of other antidepressants.	→ There are guidelines regarding safe switching of antidepressants, as time intervals must occur between stopping and starting MAOIs and other antidepressants.

Other antidepressants

Examples	• Venlafaxine, mirtazapine	
Mode of action	• Venlafaxine inhibits serotonin and noradrenaline re-uptake • Mirtazapine inhibits presynaptic a$_2$-adrenoceptors • Common for these drugs is that they inhibit monoamine reuptake	
Route of delivery	• PO	
Indications	• Treatment of major depressive disorders following unsuccessful treatment with SSRIs • Generalized anxiety disorder (venlafaxine) • Panic disorder, with or without agoraphobia	→ Mirtazapine is particularly useful in improving sleep in depressed patients with insomnia and it can also increase appetite
Cautions and contraindications	• Venlafaxine should be avoided in pregnancy but mirtazapine can be used • Cardiac arrhythmias and uncontrolled hypertension (venlafaxine) • Dose reduction with venlafaxine in hepatic impairment, but mirtazapine should be used with caution in hepatic impairment	→ Risk of neonatal effects → High risk of cardiac arrhythmias and uncontrolled HTN
Monitoring	• Review patient to check if drug has helped to improve mood • Measure blood pressure throughout treatment in patients with cardiovascular disease • If confusion or falls occur, check U+Es or serum sodium to exclude hyponatraemia	
Interactions	• NSAIDs, anticoagulants, antiplatelet drugs, SSRIs • MAOIs	→ Increased risk of bleeding → Increased risk of CNS toxicity

Side-effects	• Common or very common:
	  – GI upset e.g. abdominal pain, nausea, vomiting, diarrhoea, flatulence
	  – Rashes
	  – Fatigue
	  – Headache
	  – Hypertension
	  – Visual disturbances
	  – Dry mouth
	  – Weight changes
	  – Anxiety and nervousness
	  – Dizziness
	  – Withdrawal symptoms (especially with venlafaxine)	

Other antidepressants – *cont'd*		

Side-effects – **cont'd**	• Uncommon, rare, very rare or frequency not known:
	  – Arrhythmias
	  – Bleeding disorders
	  – Postural hypotension
	  – QT interval prolongation with venlafaxine
	  – Neuroleptic malignant syndrome
	  – Angle-closure glaucoma	

Patient counselling	• ***Impairment of normal abilities:*** • ***Withdrawal symptoms:***	➤ Warn the patient that the drug can cause drowsiness that may impair their ability to drive or operate machinery. ➤ If drug is withdrawn too abruptly, the patient may suffer from withdrawal symptoms such as headache, anxiety, tremor, GI disturbances, paraesthesia, sleep disturbances and sweating. It is recommended to withdraw drug gradually over several weeks.

Lithium

Examples	• Lithium citrate, lithium carbonate	→ Contain different concentrations of lithium so it is important to keep the patient on the same formulation throughout treatment → Must be prescribed by brand, not generically
Mode of action	• Lithium modifies the production and turnover of certain neurotransmitters, particularly serotonin, and may also block dopamine receptors • Lithium alters concentrations of certain electrolytes and may reduce thyroid activity	→ Exact mechanism of action unknown
Routes of delivery	• PO	
Indications	• Acute episodes of mania and hypomania • Recurrent depression where treatment with other antidepressants has failed • Bipolar affective disorder • Control of aggressive behaviour or intentional self-harm	
Cautions and contraindications	• Contraindicated in cardiac disease, personal or family history of Brugada syndrome, untreated hypothyroidism (lithium therapy can cause or exacerbate hypothyroidism) and in breastfeeding (lithium is present in breast milk) • Use with caution in pregnancy • Patients with low body sodium levels e.g. dehydrated, taking low sodium diet	→ Risk of fetal cardiac malformation (Epstein's anomaly); only consider lithium if benefit outweighs risk → Increased risk of lithium toxicity
Interactions	• Increased serum-lithium concentration: – Diuretics – ACEi, ARBs and NSAIDs • Reduced serum-lithium concentration: – Sodium chloride supplements • QT prolongation: – Amiodarone, venlafaxine • Increased risk of torsade de pointes: – Aminophylline, clarithromycin • Increased risk of serotonin syndrome – SSRIs, MAOIs	→ Sodium depletion, 2° to diuretics, increases toxicity → Reduce lithium clearance as these drugs affect renal function
Monitoring	• **Narrow therapeutic window and high toxicity risk** • Monitor plasma lithium levels, which should be 0.4–1 mmol/L • When starting lithium, measure patient's weight and check FBC, U+Es, TFTs, eGFR and obtain an ECG. Check serum lithium levels 1 week after initiation of therapy and after every dose adjustment (NICE 2014, CG185) • Note that blood lithium levels should be checked 12 hours after last dose	

Lithium – *cont'd*

Monitoring – **cont'd**	• Check renal function every 6 months • Annual measurement of BP, weight and body mass index (BMI) • A shared-care plan should be established with the patient's GP	→ Lithium is excreted by the kidneys → If the patient's weight increases significantly during lithium treatment, consider weight management strategies to avoid adverse effects on patient's health
Side-effects	• Common: – Fine tremor – Thirst – Polyuria and diabetes insipidus – Weight gain – Taste disturbance (metallic taste in the mouth) – Hypothyroidism – Goitre • Rare: – Lithium toxicity	• Mnemonic **LITHIUM (lithium side-effects)** **L**eucocytosis (rare) **I**nsipidus (diabetes) **T**remors **H**ypothyroidism **I**ncreased weight (weight gain) **U**rine excess **M**ums beware (teratogenic) → Signs of lithium toxicity include anorexia, nausea, vomiting, nystagmus, coarse tremor, dysarthria, ataxia and in severe cases, loss of consciousness, seizures and death (*Psychiatry: a clinical handbook*, Azam *et al.*, 2016)
Patient counselling	• *Why and how to take lithium:* • *Stay hydrated and do not make dietary changes:* • *Non-compliance and risk of relapse:* • *Blood tests:* • *Signs of lithium toxicity:*	→ Lithium works as a mood stabilizer and it is advisable that lithium therapy is not started unless there is an intention to continue for 3 years because poor compliance may precipitate rebound mania or hypomania (*Psychiatry* 3rd edition, Burton, 2016). Lithium should be taken at the same time each day and the patient should not take more than the prescribed dose. → It is important to maintain an adequate fluid intake and to avoid dietary changes that reduce or increase sodium intake. → It is important that the patient does not stop taking lithium unless advised by a doctor. If the patient stops taking lithium suddenly there is a risk of relapse. → At the start of treatment the patient will have regular blood tests to ensure that the level of lithium in the blood is sufficient, as lithium has a narrow therapeutic range and there is a high risk of toxicity if the patient's dose is incorrect. → The patient should be aware of and vigilant about signs of lithium toxicity such as anorexia, nausea, vomiting, nystagmus, coarse tremor, dysarthria, ataxia, loss of consciousness and seizures. It is important to seek medical help immediately if lithium toxicity is suspected.

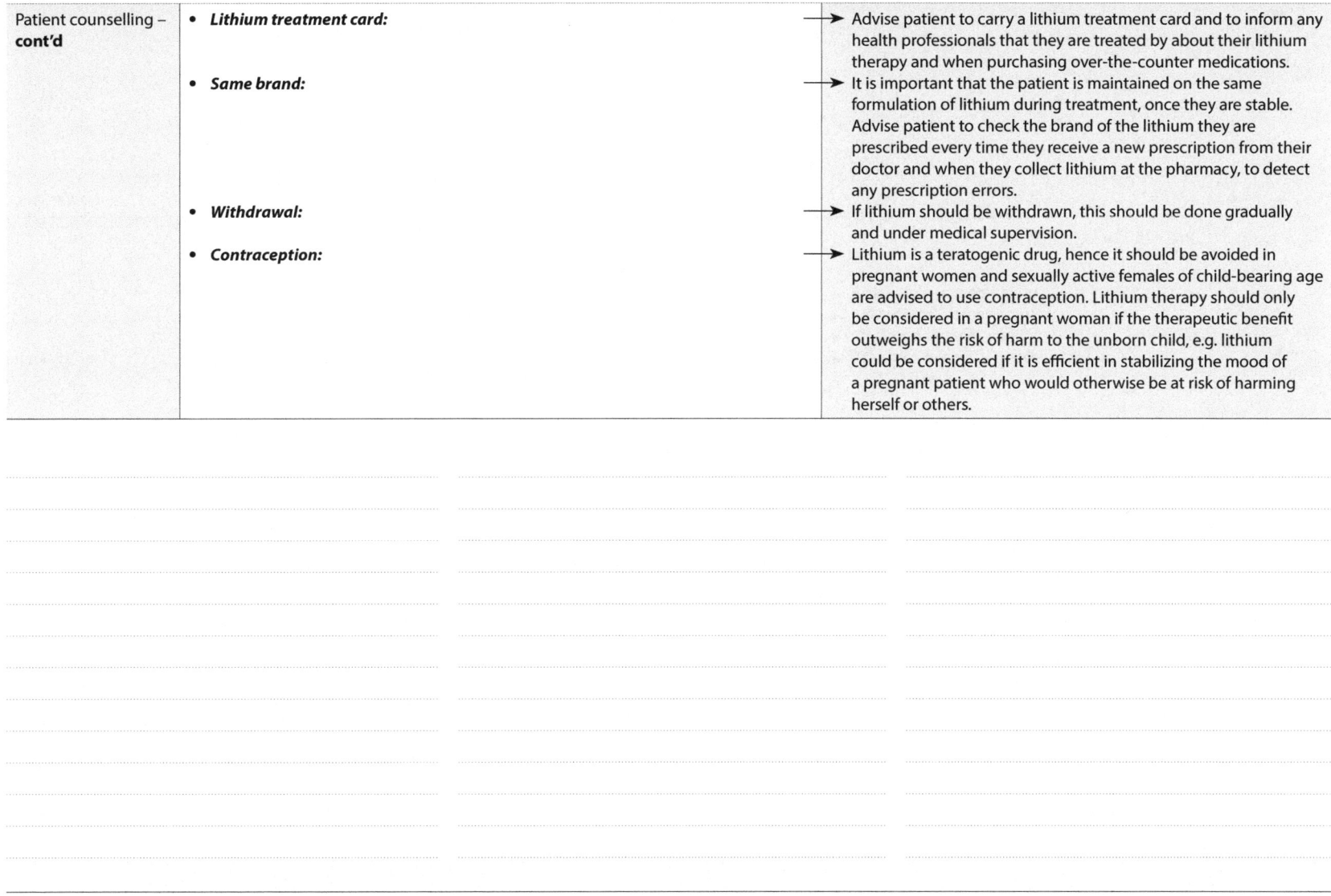

Patient counselling – **cont'd**	• **Lithium treatment card:**	→	Advise patient to carry a lithium treatment card and to inform any health professionals that they are treated by about their lithium therapy and when purchasing over-the-counter medications.
	• **Same brand:**	→	It is important that the patient is maintained on the same formulation of lithium during treatment, once they are stable. Advise patient to check the brand of the lithium they are prescribed every time they receive a new prescription from their doctor and when they collect lithium at the pharmacy, to detect any prescription errors.
	• **Withdrawal:**	→	If lithium should be withdrawn, this should be done gradually and under medical supervision.
	• **Contraception:**	→	Lithium is a teratogenic drug, hence it should be avoided in pregnant women and sexually active females of child-bearing age are advised to use contraception. Lithium therapy should only be considered in a pregnant woman if the therapeutic benefit outweighs the risk of harm to the unborn child, e.g. lithium could be considered if it is efficient in stabilizing the mood of a pregnant patient who would otherwise be at risk of harming herself or others.

Benzodiazepines		
Examples	• Diazepam, temazepam, lorazepam, chlordiazepoxide	
Mode of action	• Increase affinity of the inhibitory neurotransmitter GABA to bind to the GABA$_A$ receptor – this causes post-synaptic chloride ion channels to open	
Route of delivery	• PO, IM, IV, buccal or rectal administration	→ Resuscitation facilities must be available when administering IV benzodiazepines
Indications	• Treatment of seizures and status epilepticus • Short-term treatment for severe, distressing or disabling anxiety • Short-term treatment for insomnia • Procedural sedation • Alcohol withdrawal (chlordiazepoxide) • Tetanus, muscle spasm, acute drug-induced dystonic reactions (diazepam)	
Cautions and contraindications	• Contraindicated in respiratory depression, respiratory failure and neuromuscular conditions, e.g. unstable myasthenia gravis • Avoid in liver failure • Consider lower doses in elderly patients or avoid (if possible)	→ In overdose, benzodiazepines can cause a loss of airway reflexes, which can lead to airway obstruction, and patients with respiratory or neuromuscular problems are at an increased risk → Risk of provoking hepatic encephalopathy → More susceptible to benzodiazepine side-effects
Monitoring	• Monitor vital signs and clinical state frequently when administering drug IV or in high oral doses • Ask about symptoms and side-effects when reviewing patients who take benzodiazepines in the community	
Interactions	• CYP450 inhibitors • Alcohol and opioids • Antihypertensive medications • Clozapine • Flumazenil should not be administered following use of diazepam to treat seizures, due to the risk of intractable seizures (Richards and Aronson, *Oxford Handbook of Practical Drug Therapy*, 2005, p. 267)	→ Increased effects of benzodiazepines → Increased sedative effects → Increased hypotensive effects → Increased CNS depression

Side-effects	• Common:
	  – Amnesia, confusion, drowsiness
	  – Ataxia, muscle weakness
	  – Dependence
	• Uncommon:
	  – GI disturbances
	  – Visual disturbances, headache, dizziness, tremor, dysarthria
	  – Changes in libido, gynaecomastia	

Side-effects – **cont'd**	• Rare or frequency not known: – Apnoea, respiratory depression, blood disorders, jaundice, hypotension, hallucinations, changes in mood and behaviour (note that benzodiazepine use can cause rebound agitation)	
Patient counselling	• *For short-term use only:*	→ Inform patients that benzodiazepines are a short-term treatment and not a long-term solution to a patient's problems and that they are highly addictive. Benzodiazepines should not be taken for more than 4 weeks and they should not be taken every day.
	• *Impairment of normal abilities:*	→ Warn the patient that the benzodiazepine can cause drowsiness that may impair their ability to drive or operate machinery. Patients who receive benzodiazepines for procedural sedation should be informed that they should not drive afterwards.
	• *Withdrawal effects:*	→ Benzodiazepines are very addictive and they can cause withdrawal symptoms when they are stopped.
	• *Stop alcohol consumption whilst on chlordiazepoxide:*	→ Patients who take chlordiazepoxide for alcohol withdrawal should be informed that they must stop drinking alcohol whilst taking this drug.

Antipsychotics

Examples	**Antipsychotics can be subdivided into typical (1st generation) and atypical (2nd generation) antipsychotics**	
	• Typical antipsychotics: chlorpromazine, prochlorperazine and haloperidol	→ Older antipsychotic medications that are less commonly prescribed due to their increased risk of extrapyramidal side-effects
	• Atypical antipsychotics: risperidone, quetiapine, olanzapine and clozapine	→ Atypical antipsychotics prescribed 1st line in schizophrenia
		→ Clozapine should only be prescribed if treatment with two or more antipsychotics has failed (NICE 2014, CG178)
Mode of action	• Block post-synaptic dopamine D_2-receptors in the brain and thus increase dopamine levels	→ Note that typical antipsychotics are non-specific and they affect other receptors in addition to dopamine D_2-receptors, hence the wide range of side-effects
Routes of delivery	• PO, IM, S/C	→ The Royal College of Psychiatrists has issued guidance stating that the doses higher than those stated in the BNF are unlicensed and it advises considering alternative options before prescribing unlicensed doses (BNF 2017)
	• Before starting a patient on an antipsychotic as a depot injection, the patient should be given a test dose (NICE 2014, CG178)	
Indications	• Schizophrenia	
	• Bipolar disorder	
	• Agitation and restlessness in the elderly	→ Review each patient clinically before prescribing an antipsychotic for agitation and investigate the cause of their agitation
Cautions and contraindications	• Typical antipsychotics are contraindicated in Parkinson's disease due to extrapyramidal side-effects	
	• Clozapine should be used with caution in cardiovascular disease	
	• Avoid in dementia	→ Dementia and use of antipsychotics has been correlated with a higher risk of stroke and death
	• Use with caution in elderly people	→ More susceptible to antipsychotic side-effects
Interactions	• Amiodarone, macrolides, SSRIs, quinine	→ Increased risk of QT interval prolongation
	• Alcohol, opioids	→ Sedation and increased CNS effects
	• Clozapine interacts with carbamazepine	→ Increased risk of agranulocytosis
	• Grapefruit juice may increase exposure to quetiapine (BNF, 2017)	
Monitoring	• Before an antipsychotic is started, measurement of weight, waist circumference, pulse rate and blood pressure should be checked and an assessment of the patient's general health, including blood tests, should be performed; the doctor may also wish to obtain an ECG (NICE 2014, CG178)	→ There is a risk of metabolic disturbances being caused by antipsychotics, thus a baseline assessment of the patient's general health should be undertaken
	• For patients starting clozapine: monitor FBC weekly for 18 weeks, then fortnightly until 1 year; after 1 year monitor FBC every 4 weeks	→ Clozapine causes agranulocytosis in 1% of patients (*Psychiatry* 3rd edition, Burton, 2016)
		→ Discontinue clozapine immediately if WCC $<1.5 \times 10^4$ (or as indicated by local guidelines)

Monitoring – **cont'd**	• Some antipsychotics require monitoring of prolactin concentration at the start of therapy, at 6 months, and then yearly	→ Consider prolactin monitoring in patients who show signs of hyperprolactinaemia, even if this adverse effect is not commonly associated with their antipsychotic drug

Side-effects	• General side-effects:
	  – Sedation
	  – Extrapyramidal side-effects
	  – Weight gain, hypertension, diabetes mellitus, hypercholesterolaemia and sexual dysfunction
	• Specific side-effects:
	  – Neutropenia, agranulocytosis (clozapine)
	  – Gynaecomastia and galactorrhoea (risperidone)
		→ Beneficial in agitated patients but use with caution
		
		→ Warn patients of these side-effects in advance as they are unwanted effects that may cause non-adherence
		
		→ Increased prolactin secretion with risperidone use

Patient counselling	• ***Counselling on choice of antipsychotic:*** • ***Pregnancy and breastfeeding:***	→ Prior to starting antipsychotic medication, the doctor should discuss different options for antipsychotic drugs with the patient and explain the benefits, risks and side-effects of each drug. The patient should be asked which side-effects they are willing to accept and they should be involved in the final decision of which antipsychotic to start (NICE 2014, CG178). Furthermore, it is important to emphasize the importance of compliance with the drug and of the patient attending follow-up appointments. → According to the BNF, there have been reports of extrapyramidal side-effects and withdrawal symptoms in the neonate when antipsychotic medications have been taken in the 3rd trimester. In instances where maternal use in the 3rd trimester has occurred, neonates must be monitored for respiratory distress and CNS effects such as agitation and hypotonia. Antipsychotics should be avoided in breastfeeding due to a lack of information confirming short- and long-term safety.

Anti-epileptics

Examples	• Carbamazepine, lamotrigine, levetiracetam, pregabalin, gabapentin, sodium valproate • Phenytoin is covered under *Emergency Drugs* in *Chapter 15* Note that carbamazepine should be prescribed by brand	➤ Anti-epileptic drugs are prescribed under brand name and it is essential that patients be maintained on the same brand and same formulation during their treatment ➤ Ensure that you are aware of the specific indication and formulation before prescribing an anti-epileptic drug
Mode of action	Anti-epileptic medications result in reduced seizure activity through different mechanisms: • Lamotrigine and sodium valproate block voltage-gated Na^+ channels to reduce neurotransmission • Carbamazepine slows recovery of voltage-gated Na^+ channels, opens potassium channels and releases GABA • Pregabalin, gabapentin and levetiracetam have an unknown mode of action	
Routes of delivery	• PO, IV	
Indications	• Epilepsy, trigeminal neuralgia and prophylaxis of bipolar disorder (carbamazepine) • Monotherapy in focal, generalized and absence seizures, prophylaxis of depressive episodes in bipolar disorder (lamotrigine) • Partial seizures (levetiracetam) • Partial seizures, neuropathic pain and generalized anxiety disorders (pregabalin and gabapentin) • All types of epilepsy (sodium valproate)	
Cautions and contraindications	• Sodium valproate and lamotrigine are contraindicated in pregnancy • Levetiracetam should be avoided in pregnancy unless benefit outweighs risk • Carbamazepine and pregabalin may be used with caution in pregnancy • Parkinson's disease and myoclonic seizures • Caution in renal and hepatic impairment	➤ May be exacerbated by lamotrigine ➤ Carbamazepine should be withdrawn immediately if liver function deteriorates or if acute liver disease occurs ➤ Sodium valproate should be avoided in active liver disease and hepatic impairment
Monitoring	• General: ask about seizure activity and side-effects of anti-epileptic drug when reviewing patient • Carbamazepine: check U+Es (if confusion or falls occur) and monitor plasma carbamazepine levels (target 4–10 mg/L) • Sodium valproate: check baseline FBC and repeat FBC before any invasive procedures, check baseline LFTs and then repeat LFTs every 6 months	➤ To assess whether seizure activity is reduced by anti-epileptic drug and whether drug is well tolerated by patient ➤ To exclude hyponatraemia ➤ Sodium valproate can cause blood dyscrasias ➤ Sodium valproate is dangerous in liver disease and liver impairment
Interactions	• CNS depressants e.g. opioids, benzodiazepines and alcohol (lamotrigine, pregabalin, levetiracetam) • Antidepressants and St John's wort (lamotrigine)	➤ Increased risk of CNS depression ➤ Plasma concentration of lamotrigine is reduced, hence dose adjustment required

Interactions – **cont'd**	• Clozapine (carbamazepine) • Combined hormonal contraceptives (lamotrigine) • Statins, alcohol, paracetamol, tetracyclines, carbapenems (sodium valproate) • Anticonvulsants can interact with each other	→ Increased risk of agranulocytosis → Altered exposure to lamotrigine → Increased risk of hepatotoxicity *Please note that interactions between anti-epileptic medications are complex and unpredictable, and they may increase toxicity without an increased therapeutic effect. The most common cause of interactions is hepatic enzyme induction or inhibition.*

Side-effects	• General:
	  – Nausea, vomiting
	  – Dizziness, diplopia, blurred vision, ataxia
	  – Hyponatraemia
	  – Teratogenicity
	  – All anti-epileptic medications are associated with a small increased risk of suicidal thoughts and behaviour (MHRA 2008)
	• Specific:
	  – Weight gain, pancreatitis, thrombocytopenia (sodium valproate)
	  – Cardiac conduction disturbances, leucopenia, Stevens–Johnson syndrome (carbamazepine)
	  – Weight gain, hypertension, leucopenia (pregabalin)
	  – Drowsiness, nausea, vomiting, diarrhoea, dyspepsia, anorexia (levetiracetam)
		• Mnemonic **VALPROATE (sodium valproate side-effects)**
		Vomiting
		Alopecia
		Liver dysfunction
		Pancreatitis
		Retention of fat (weight gain)
		Oedema
		Anorexia
		Teratogenicity, tremor
		Enzyme inhibition

Patient counselling	• ***Adverse side-effects:*** • ***Do not stop taking drug unless advised by a doctor:*** • ***Many anti-epileptic drugs are teratogenic:*** • ***Beware of medications and triggers to epilepsy:*** • ***UK Epilepsy and Pregnancy Register:***	→ Inform patient of adverse effects specific to their anti-epileptic drug and of signs to look out for. → Inform patients that it is not advisable to stop using their anti-epileptic drug unless advised by a doctor. It is important that anti-epileptic drugs are withdrawn gradually. → Warn female patients of child-bearing age that their anti-epileptic drug may cause harm to an unborn child; thus reliable contraception should be used in women who do not wish to conceive. It is not recommended that certain anti-epileptic drugs, e.g. sodium valproate, be used in women wishing to conceive, therefore women who are planning to become pregnant should inform the doctor managing their epilepsy immediately when they decide to try to conceive. Folic acid should be taken pre-conception and during pregnancy. → Certain medications and substances may lower the seizure threshold. If known, they should be avoided or used with caution in the epileptic patient. → All pregnant women with epilepsy are encouraged to notify the UK Epilepsy and Pregnancy Register.

Anti-epileptics – *cont'd*

| Patient counselling – **cont'd** | • *Sudden unexpected death in Epilepsy (SUDEP):* | → If someone with epilepsy dies suddenly and unexpectedly, and no obvious cause of death can be found, it is called sudden unexpected death in epilepsy (SUDEP). Premature death in people with epilepsy is higher than in the general population, and SUDEP is the most common cause of this. SUDEP has been shown to be connected with seizures, particularly tonic-clonic (convulsive) seizures. The exact cause is not known and there may be no single explanation. However, it is thought that seizure activity in the brain may sometimes cause changes in the person's heartbeat or breathing. This could cause the person to stop breathing or their heart to stop beating. Cases of SUDEP should be reported and support should be made available to affected families (Epilepsy Action, April 2016). |

Ways to reduce the risks of SUDEP if you have epilepsy:

Seizure control: the most effective way to reduce the risk of SUDEP is to have as few seizures as possible. If your seizures are not controlled, here are some ways to manage your epilepsy:

- Always take your epilepsy medicines exactly as prescribed
- Never stop taking your epilepsy medicines, or make changes to them, without talking to your doctor first
- Make sure you never run out of your epilepsy medicines
- Ask your epilepsy specialist or epilepsy nurse in advance what you should do if you ever forget to take your epilepsy medicines
- Ask to be referred to an epilepsy specialist for a review of your epilepsy. They may be able to suggest changes to your epilepsy medicines, or other treatment options, which may include surgery
- Try not to sleep on your stomach as recent research suggests that people with epilepsy who sleep on their stomach may be at higher risk of SUDEP

Other possible helpful ideas:

- **Keep a diary of your seizures.** This can help doctors when they are considering the best treatment for you. It may also help you to see if there is a pattern to your seizures.
- **Avoid situations which may trigger your seizures.** Common triggers include forgotten epilepsy medicines, lack of sleep, stress and too much alcohol.
- **Consider buying a safety pillow.** Safety pillows have small holes. They may help you breathe more easily than a normal pillow if you are lying face down during a seizure. There is no evidence, however, that safety pillows reduce the risk of SUDEP.
- If your seizures happen at night, talk to your family doctor or epilepsy specialist nurse about using a **bed alarm**. Bed alarms can alert another person if you have a seizure. This will help the person to help you. For example, they can put you in the recovery position or call for an ambulance, if necessary. (Be aware that bed alarms can be very expensive and are not always perfect. They may sometimes miss seizures or go off without a reason. And it's important to know that there is no proof that bed alarms reduce the risk of SUDEP.) `
- **Tell people about your epilepsy** and let them know how they can help you if you have a tonic-clonic seizure. You may choose to wear identity jewellery or carry some form of epilepsy awareness card to make other people aware of your epilepsy.

(Epilepsy Action, April 2016; see website for more information www.epilepsy.org.uk/info/sudep-sudden-unexpected-death-in-epilepsy)

Xanthine oxidase inhibitors

Examples	• Allopurinol, feboxustat	
Mode of action	• Prevents xanthine from being oxidized to uric acid by competitively inhibiting the enzyme xanthine oxidase	→ Lowering uric acid levels that are excessive helps reduce severity of gout and reduces the likelihood of uric acid kidney stones
Routes of delivery	• PO, IV	
Indications	• Prophylaxis of gout attacks in patients with chronic gout • Prophylaxis of uric acid kidney stones • Prophylaxis of hyperuricaemia associated with chemotherapy	
Cautions and contraindications	• Contraindicated in acute gout	→ Patients must not be started on allopurinol until acute attack resolves
Interactions	• Warfarin • Theophylline • ACEi and thiazide diuretics • Amoxicillin • Azathioprine	→ Increased effect of warfarin as its metabolism is reduced → Possible increase in serum levels of theophylline → Increased risk of hypersensitivity → Increased risk of skin rash → Enhanced effect and increased risk of toxicity of azathioprine
Monitoring	• Careful monitoring required due to concerns with hypersensitivity reactions: check uric acid levels, FBC and LFTs	

Side-effects	• Common:
	  – Gastrointestinal upset
	  – Rashes
	• Less common:
	  – Hypersensitivity reactions
	  – Blood disorders
	  – Hepatotoxicity
	  – Seizures (very rare)
		→ BNF advises to withdraw drug but reintroduce drug cautiously if the rash was mild, but drug should be discontinued promptly if rash recurs

Patient counselling	• ***Do not prescribe to hypersensitive patients:*** • ***When to seek help:*** • ***Not for acute gout:*** • ***Stay hydrated:***	→ Confirm that the patient has not had a severe allergic reaction to allopurinol before prescribing this drug. → Warn the patient to seek medical help urgently if they notice a rash, swelling of the lips or face, yellowing of the eyes or skin, painful urination or blood in the urine. → Ensure that the patient is aware that allopurinol should not be used during acute gout attacks. Xanthine oxidase inhibitors are normally started at least 1–2 weeks after a gout attack has settled. → Drink plenty of fluids when taking allopurinol

P-glycoprotein substrates

Examples	• Colchicine	
Mode of action	• Binds to microtubular protein tubulin in neutrophils, inhibiting immune response • Inhibits release of histamine mast cells	➤ These changes reduce the immune response that is mounted during an acute gout attack
Route of delivery	• PO	
Indications	• Treatment of acute gout attacks • Short-term prophylaxis of gout • Familial Mediterranean fever (FMF)	➤ To be used as an alternative to NSAIDs ➤ Unlicensed use
Cautions and contraindications	• Contraindicated in colchicine hypersensitivity, blood dyscrasias, pregnancy and breastfeeding • Use with caution in elderly patients and those with severe disorders of the cardiovascular, gastrointestinal, renal or hepatic systems	➤ Similar to patients with renal or hepatic impairment, elderly patients struggle to clear colchicine
Monitoring	• Monitor patient for adverse effects	
Interactions	• Grapefruit juice, macrolide antibiotics, antifungal agents, rate-limiting CCBs, amiodarone, digoxin • Ciclosporin • Statins and fibrates	➤ May increase risk of colchicine toxicity – reduce colchicine by half when used concomitantly with moderate CYP3A4 inhibitors ➤ May increase risk of nephrotoxicity and colchicine toxicity ➤ May increase risk of myopathy

Side-effects	• Common:
	   – Abdominal pain
	   – Nausea
	   – Vomiting
	 • Less common:
	   – Alopecia
	   – Blood disorders
	   – Myopathy
	   – Peripheral neuritis
	
	 • Frequency not known:
	   – Rash
	   – GI bleeding
	   – Diarrhoea (if excessive doses taken)
	   – Renal impairment	

Patient counselling	• ***Hypersensitivity status:*** • ***Used in acute gout:*** • ***Avoid grapefruit juice:*** • ***Lifestyle measures:***	➤ Confirm patient is not hypersensitive to colchicine before prescribing it. ➤ Clarify that patient understands that colchicine should be used for acute attacks (not allopurinol), and is normally taken in short courses. ➤ Do not consume grapefruit juice when taking colchicine. ➤ Advise the patient regarding lifestyle measures to reduce gout, e.g. weight loss, healthy diet.

Methotrexate

Examples	• Methotrexate	
Mode of action	• Folic acid antagonist: prevents cellular replication by inhibiting dihydrofolate reductase, an enzyme which converts folic acid to tetrahydrofolate (required for DNA replication) • Acts directly on RNA and protein synthesis	
Routes of delivery	• PO	→ **Once weekly dosing** – prescribing methotrexate more frequently than once a week is a Never Event → Comes in tablet form in two doses, 2.5 mg and 10 mg → It is recommended that only 2.5 mg tablets are prescribed to avoid drug errors with methotrexate
Indications	• Malignant disease (as part of chemotherapy) • Rheumatoid arthritis • Severe psoriasis • Crohn's disease • Medical management of ectopic pregnancy	→ Unlicensed indication
Cautions and contraindications	• Acute porphyrias • Pregnancy • Breastfeeding • Immunodeficiency syndromes (non-malignant) • Active infections (non-malignant) • Ascites and significant pleural effusions • Avoid in hepatic impairment and reduce dose in renal impairment – nephrotoxic at high doses • Use with caution in photosensitivity	→ Consider performing a pregnancy test to exclude pregnancy before starting methotrexate → Methotrexate can accumulate into these tissue fluids and, if present, they should be drained before methotrexate treatment

Interactions	• Increased risk of methotrexate toxicity due to reduced elimination of drug:
	  – Aspirin
	  – NSAIDs
	  – Penicillins
	  – Ciprofloxacin
	• Increased risk of haematological toxicity:
	  – Corticosteroids
	  – Trimethoprim
	  – Co-trimoxazole
	• Increased risk of agranulocytosis:
	  – Clozapine	

Monitoring	• **Narrow therapeutic window and high toxicity risk**	→ Frequent monitoring required
	• Baseline FBC, U+Es and LFTs then measurements every 2 weeks until 6 weeks after dose has stabilized and then monitor FBC, U+Es and LFTs every 6–12 months afterwards (Richards and Aronson, *Oxford Handbook of Practical Drug Therapy*, 2005, p. 499)	→ To detect blood dyscrasias, liver dysfunction or renal impairment
	• Some clinicians obtain a CXR before starting methotrexate	→ If signs of pulmonary toxicity, a baseline CXR can be used for comparison with new imaging
Side-effects	• Rare: – Pneumonitis • Frequency not known: – Nausea, vomiting, diarrhoea, abdominal discomfort – Skin rashes, photosensitivity, mouth ulcers, hair loss – Pulmonary fibrosis – Bone marrow failure and other blood disorders – Infertility – Teratogenicity	→ Inform GP about skin rashes and mouth ulcers → Drug may cause infertility which may be reversible → Women and men of child-bearing age who are sexually active must use secure contraception during methotrexate treatment and for 3 months after stopping methotrexate
Patient counselling	• ***How to take:*** methotrexate is taken as a once-weekly dose and it should be taken at the same time on the same day every week (e.g. every Wednesday at 8 am). Compliance is very important. • ***How to handle tablets:*** avoid handling tablets as much as possible and wash hands afterwards. Ensure tablets are out of reach of young children. • ***Missed doses:*** contact your GP for advice. Do not take two doses together or take more than the prescribed dose, if you discover that you have missed a dose of methotrexate. • ***Folic acid supplements:*** folic acid may be co-prescribed to prevent folic acid deficiency. • ***Do not take NSAIDs over the counter:*** taking methotrexate and NSAIDs at the same time can increase the risk of nephrotoxicity. • ***Contraception:*** females of child-bearing age and all males who are sexually active whilst taking methotrexate must use secure contraception to prevent pregnancy during treatment and for 3 months after stopping treatment. • ***Infertility:*** methotrexate may cause reduced fertility, which may be reversible. • ***Inform GP about the following symptoms:*** sore throat, bruising and mouth ulcers (signs of blood disorders), nausea, vomiting, abdominal discomfort and dark urine (signs of liver toxicity), shortness of breath (respiratory compromise).	→ It is good practice to issue methotrexate treatment booklets, which contain information for patients regarding methotrexate and in which patients can record their doses and blood results

Bisphosphonates

Examples	• Alendronic acid, risedronate sodium, zoledronic acid	
Mode of action	• Reduce bone turnover by inhibiting the action of osteoclasts (which cause bone resorption) and by being absorbed into bone • Lower calcium levels by binding to calcium	
Routes of delivery	• PO, IV infusion	
Indications	• Prophylaxis and treatment of corticosteroid-induced osteoporosis • Paget's disease of bone • Osteolytic lesions and bony metastases • Hypercalcaemia of malignancy	→ All patients who are having long-term treatment with steroids must be started on a bisphosphonate to prevent osteoporosis
Cautions and contraindications	• Pregnancy • Hypocalcaemia • Severe renal impairment • Use with caution in the following conditions: oesophagitis and other upper GI disorders, active GI bleeding, atypical femoral fractures	→ Increased risk of acquiring or exacerbating oesophagitis → Bisphosphonates are excreted by the kidneys
Interactions	• Antacids, calcium salts and oral iron salts • Aminoglycosides	→ Decrease absorption of oral bisphosphonates → Concomitant use increases risk of hypocalcaemia
Monitoring	• Correct any electrolyte abnormalities before starting treatment and monitor U+Es for serum calcium and phosphate levels during treatment • DEXA scans • The MHRA advises that the need to continue bisphosphonate therapy should be reassessed periodically based on the benefits and risks to the individual concerned, particularly in patients who have been taking bisphosphonates for ≥5 years	→ To detect hypocalcaemia and/or hypophosphataemia → To check whether bone density is stable

Side-effects	• Common:
	  – Oesophagitis
	  – Hypophosphataemia and hypocalcaemia
	  – Constipation or diarrhoea
	• Less common:
	  – Atypical femoral fracture
	
	  – Osteonecrosis of the jaw
	  – Osteonecrosis of the external auditory canal
		
		→ Can occur when taking oral bisphosphonates
		→ Electrolytes should be monitored during therapy
		→ It is important to maintain an adequate fluid intake
		
		→ Advise patients to report any pain in the thigh, hip or groin during treatment (MHRA/CHM advice 2011)
		→ Advice regarding dental care must be provided (MHRA/CHM advice 2009)
		→ Rare, but consider the possibility of osteonecrosis of the auditory canal in patients who present with ear symptoms (MHRA/CHM advice 2015)

Patient counselling	• **How to take:** bisphosphonates should be taken on an empty stomach (at least 30 minutes before food or drink) and swallowed with plenty of water, and the patient needs to remain sitting or standing for 30 minutes after taking this drug to reduce gastric irritation.	→ Once-weekly dosing has been implemented to increase compliance and reduce side-effects
	• **Oesophageal dysfunction:** tell patient to inform their doctor if they experience irritation of the oesophagus, pain or difficulty with swallowing. This could be a sign of oesophagitis, which may be drug-induced.	
	• **Oral hygiene to prevent or detect osteonecrosis of the jaw:** it is important to have a dental check-up before starting treatment, and to maintain regular dental check-ups during treatment. Patients should be advised to visit their dentist before, during and after treatment (MHRA/CHM advice 2015).	
	• **Atypical femoral fractures:** although atypical femoral fractures associated with bisphosphonate use are rare, patients should be advised to report any pain in the thigh, hip or groin during treatment (MHRA/CHM advice 2011).	
	• **Ear problems:** ask patient to report any problems with the ears, such as pain, discharge and infections during treatment (MHRA/CHM advice 2015).	

Section II:

Prescribing by situation

How do you assess a patient's fluid status? *(adapted from NICE 2017, CG174, Algorithm 1: Assessment)*

History	• Does the patient think that their oral fluid intake has been sufficient? Does the patient feel thirsty? Is the patient receiving fluid through other means, e.g. NG feed, TPN? • What co-morbidities does the patient have? • Has the patient experienced any diarrhoea or vomiting? • Does the patient have any stomas or drains or other means of fluid loss?
Appearance of the skin and mucous membranes	• Do the skin or mucous membranes appear dry? • Does the patient have sunken eyes? • What is the skin turgor?
Signs of fluid overload	• Elevated JVP • Ascites • Peripheral oedema • Pulmonary oedema
Signs of hypovolaemia that may indicate that patient needs fluid resuscitation	• Systolic BP <100 mmHg • Heart rate >90 bpm • Capillary refill >2 s or peripheries cold to touch • Respiratory rate >20 breaths per min • NEWS ≥5 • 45° passive leg raising suggests fluid responsiveness
Blood pressure	• Hypotension may suggest dehydration but there are other causes of hypotension, e.g. sepsis, haemorrhage, etc. • Check for postural hypotension
Micturition	• Is the patient passing urine? • If the patient is passing urine through a catheter, how much is in the catheter bag (and has it been emptied recently)? • What colour is the urine? • If there is no urine output in a catheterized patient, it is essential to check whether the catheter is patent.
Fluid balance charts	• What do the patient's fluid balance charts reveal? Remember to look at the past days' fluid balance charts to detect a trend, in addition to the current chart. • What is the patient's urine output, compared to input? The minimum obligatory volume of urine (MOVU) output is 0.5 ml/kg/h.
Daily weights	• Has the patient's weight changed at all during their stay in hospital?
Blood results	• Review the patient's blood results, paying particular attention to the patient's urea, creatinine and electrolytes, and be prepared to act on any abnormalities. • Elevated values of urea and creatinine compared to the patient's baseline may suggest that a patient is suffering from an acute kidney injury (AKI) and the first course of action is normally to rehydrate the patient and to stop or withhold any nephrotoxic drugs.

What are the basic principles of fluid balance?

- Two-thirds of the human body consists of water. Women have slightly more adipose tissue than men, thus they contain less water. Similarly, there is a slight variation between individuals of the same gender depending on body composition and it is expected that individuals gain fat as they age.
- This water is contained in two separate compartments: the intracellular compartment (ICF) and the extracellular compartment (ECF).
- The ICF is made up of the fluid inside the cells. This is the fluid that is contained within the cell membranes and it has a high potassium concentration and a low sodium concentration.
- The ECF consists of the fluid outside the cells. It is subdivided into the interstitial compartment (75% of the ECF) and the intravascular compartment (25% of the ECF). ECF has a high sodium concentration and a low potassium concentration.
- Fluid moves between the different compartments by diffusion and there are three forces (hydrostatic pressure, osmotic pressure and oncotic pressure) that govern this movement.
- In order to maintain homeostasis, fluid input (oral fluids, IV fluids, NG feeding, TPN) must equal fluid output (urine output, faeces, stoma output, vomiting, sweat, haemorrhage).
- Intravenous fluids are prescribed for routine maintenance, fluid resuscitation and replacement of electrolytes.
- The principle is that the intravenous fluid replacing a fluid deficit should be similar in content where possible. For example, if the patient is having GI tract losses, e.g. diarrhoea and vomiting, they are losing fluid rich in sodium, chloride, potassium, bicarbonate and hydrogen ions (if vomiting up gastric content which is acidic), an appropriate fluid for replacement is Hartmann's solution, which is similar to extracellular fluid and is sometimes referred to as *physiological fluid*.

What are the daily fluid requirements for an adult?

For maintenance (keeping vital functions working), 25–30 ml/kg/day of fluids is required, containing the following electrolytes:

- Sodium 1 mmol/kg/day
- Potassium 1 mmol/kg/day
- Chloride 1 mmol/kg/day
- 50–100 g of glucose (to prevent starvation ketosis) (NICE 2017, CG174, Algorithm 3: Routine maintenance).

A general rule of thumb is that women require up to 2 litres of fluid per day and men require up to 2.5 litres of fluid per day.

Routine maintenance + replacement of losses = total amount of intravenous fluids required

Which patients require less intravenous fluid?

Intravenous fluids should be used with caution in heart failure as excessive fluid intake can result in pulmonary oedema. Similar caution should be taken when prescribing fluids to patients who are elderly or frail, as inappropriate administration of IV fluids can easily result in fluid overload.

During initial resuscitation of patients with heart failure or patients who are frail (e.g. elderly), consider giving a 250 ml bolus of 0.9% saline instead of a 500 ml bolus of 0.9% saline.

Electrolyte and glucose content in 1 L of commonly prescribed intravenous fluids					
	Sodium	**Chloride**	**Potassium**	**Glucose**	**Other electrolytes**
0.9% sodium chloride	154 mmol	154 mmol	0 mmol	0 mmol	n/a
Hartmann's solution	131 mmol	111 mmol	5 mmol	0 mmol	2 mmol calcium 29 mmol lactate
5% dextrose	n/a (5% dextrose is 50 g glucose dissolved in 1 L water)			50 g	n/a
4% dextrose/ 0.18% saline	30 mmol	30 mmol	0 mmol	40 g	n/a

What is an appropriate choice of intravenous fluid for fluid resuscitation?

If fluid challenges are to be administered to a patient, fluid boluses of a crystalloid containing sodium 130–154 ml would be appropriate (NICE 2017, CG174, Algorithm 2: Fluid resuscitation).

However, if higher volumes of fluid for resuscitation, such as several litres of IV fluid, are given, administration of 0.9% sodium chloride may cause hyperchloraemic acidosis. Therefore, a more balanced fluid such as Hartmann's solution would be more appropriate.

What steps can be taken to prescribe intravenous fluids safely?

(1) Consider whether the patient actually needs IV fluids. Are they able to drink oral fluids independently? Can anything be done to facilitate oral fluid intake? Some patients need encouragement to drink enough fluids. If there is a possibility that the patient might need to go to theatre, keep the patient nil by mouth and set up a maintenance fluid infusion.

(2) Review the most recent blood results before prescribing fluids, to ensure prescription is appropriate for patient. This prevents harmful errors such as prescribing potassium-rich fluids to a patient with hyperkalaemia.

(3) Consider patient's co-morbidities when choosing which type of intravenous fluid to prescribe and what volume of fluid to administer. For example, if the patient has a background of heart failure or is showing signs of fluid overload, stop or reduce the volume of IV fluids prescribed.

(4) Review local guidelines or consult a senior if you are unsure which type of IV fluid to prescribe in view of a patient's physical state.

Clinical assessment of oxygenation	
Airway	• The first step of the ABCDE assessment, undertaken before history and physical examination, is to ensure that the patient has a patent airway. A patient who is alert and speaking in full sentences will have a patent airway, whereas a patient with a GCS ≤7 is at high risk of airway compromise (the reduced level of consciousness may result in the patient being unable to maintain their airway independently) and an airway adjunct should be considered.
History	• Take a history to elicit the cause of the present illness • Enquire about respiratory symptoms such as shortness of breath, shortness of breath on exertion, paroxysmal nocturnal dyspnoea, presence of productive cough and haemoptysis

Physical examination	• Pay attention to the patient's mental state; lack of oxygen perfusion can result in confusion
	• Observe the patient:
	  – Does the patient look centrally or peripherally cyanosed?
	  – Is the patient making sounds suggestive of airway obstruction e.g. stridor, gurgling, choking, snoring, wheezing or hoarseness of voice?
	  – Are there any signs of increased work of breathing e.g. use of accessory muscles or paradoxical chest movements?
	  – Does the chest wall have a normal appearance?
	  – Is the patient breathing slowly or rapidly, and does the patient appear comfortable or distressed?
	• Palpate the trachea:
	  – Is the trachea central or deviated?
	• Test chest expansion:
	  – Is chest expansion symmetrical?
	• Percuss the chest:
	  – Does the chest sound dull, resonant or hyperresonant?
	• Auscultate the chest:
	  – Is there good air entry?
	  – Are breath sounds present bilaterally and are they equal on both sides?
	  – Any added sounds present?

Oxygen saturations (SpO$_2$)	• Aim for target saturations of 94–98% in patients without COPD and 88–92% in patients with COPD until an ABG has been performed. COPD patients who do not retain CO_2 may tolerate higher oxygen saturations. • Specify the appropriate target saturation for each patient on their oxygen prescription chart (*BTS Guideline for Oxygen Use in Adults in Healthcare and Emergency Settings*, June 2017)
Respiratory rate (RR)	• Respiratory rate is the single best measure of severe illness (*BTS Guideline for Oxygen Use in Adults in Healthcare and Emergency Settings*, June 2017)
Arterial blood gas (ABG)	• The arterial blood gas is an accurate measurement of oxygenation and acid–base disturbances • It is particularly useful to obtain an ABG in critically unwell patients and in patients at risk of hypercapnoea • However, obtaining an ABG is a painful procedure and care should be taken to avoid performing ABGs on patients when not indicated
Chest X-ray (CXR)	• Consider a chest X-ray if further clinical information is needed
Other investigations	• Peak expiratory flow measurement (PEFR) and spirometry can be used to assess severity of obstructive and restrictive airway disease

In which situations should oxygen therapy be prescribed?

- The most common reason for prescribing oxygen in hospital is for treatment of patients with hypoxaemia (PaO_2 <8 kPa) or patients that are acutely unwell.
- Oxygen is normally prescribed for use in the community to manage chronic conditions, e.g. long-term oxygen therapy for COPD and palliation for lung malignancy.

Common methods of administering oxygen at ward level:

Oxygen delivery device and FiO_2	Advantages	Disadvantages
Nasal cannulae 1–4 L at FiO_2 0.28–0.36 **Note:** high flow nasal cannulae exist which provide an FiO_2 up to 0.6 and can provide humidified oxygen	Suitable in mild hypoxia Tolerated by many patients	Low amount of O_2 can be delivered Precise control of FiO_2 not possible Can cause dryness of nasal mucosa resulting in irritation or nosebleeds
Non-rebreathable mask 4–15 L at FiO_2 0.6 **Note:** FiO_2 can be increased to 0.85 with a reservoir bag and to 1.0 with a bag valve resuscitator	Does not deliver a specific FiO_2 Reservoir bag can be added to allow rebreathing	A tight seal of the mask is required to prevent air leaks
Venturi masks FiO_2 0.24–0.36	Useful in patients dependent on hypoxic respiratory drive as a fixed amount of O_2 will be administered	Re-breathing does not occur
BiPAP (bilevel positive airway pressure)	Useful in COPD and atelectasis	BiPAP is delivered using a face mask, which should fit firmly onto the patient's face; some patients may find it uncomfortable or claustrophobic
CPAP (continuous positive airway pressure)	Provides constant positive airway pressure, hence CPAP is used in heart failure and obstructive sleep apnoea to keep airways open	

Important information about home oxygen:

- Patients who require long-term oxygen therapy to manage severe breathlessness due to COPD can be prescribed home oxygen, which is contained in cylinders. These cylinders should be maintained upright and should remain at least 2 metres away from flames at all times.
- Patients must be notified of the dangers of smoking, using cookers and lighting candles, lanterns or fires whilst home oxygen is attached, as this is a fire hazard.
- If the patient experiences dryness to their lips and nose, they can use a water-based moisturizer. Petroleum-based products such as Vaseline and ointments must not be used as they can plug the air holes and serve as a fire hazard, causing chemical burns.
- Patients should be encouraged to quit smoking, as there is a reduction in clinical benefit of home oxygen in COPD patients who continue to smoke.

Penicillins

Examples	• Amoxicillin, ampicillin, flucloxacillin, benzylpenicillin, phenoxymethylpenicillin (penicillin V), piperacillin	→ End in -cillin
	• Co-amoxiclav	→ Do not forget that co-amoxiclav contains a penicillin when prescribing to a penicillin-allergic patient
Mode of action	• Inhibit cross-linking of peptide chains in the peptidoglycan bacterial cell wall, resulting in lysis of the weakened bacterial cell wall and subsequent cell death	→ Broad spectrum: effective in treating Gram +ve and Gram −ve bacteria, depending on indication → **Avoid over-prescribing of antibiotics (e.g. prescribing antibiotics when not indicated)** → **The rise of antibiotic-resistant bacteria is a serious challenge worldwide**
Route of delivery	• PO, IV, IM	→ Use sugar-free suspensions in children
Indications	• Respiratory tract infection, urinary tract infection (UTI), otitis media (amoxicillin and ampicillin) • Cellulitis (flucloxacillin) • Bacterial meningitis (benzylpenicillin) • ENT infections (phenoxymethylpenicillin) • Extended spectrum for severe infections and *Pseudomonas* (piperacillin) • Due to immunosuppression, splenectomy patients require long-term prophylactic antibiotics, usually a low-dose penicillin	→ Splenectomy patients also require further vaccinations including the annual flu jab
Cautions and contraindications	• Contra-indicated in patients with hypersensitivity reaction to penicillin • Patients with a history of immediate hypersensitivity to penicillins may also react to the cephalosporins and other beta-lactam antibiotics, so they should not receive these antibiotics (BNF 2017)	→ Always clarify details of allergic reaction to confirm that this is a true penicillin allergy
Monitoring	• Monitor WCC and C-reactive protein (CRP), review patient's clinical state	→ If starting patient on IV antibiotics, this route should be reviewed within 48 hours of starting treatment
Interactions	• Warfarin • Methotrexate	→ Some penicillins may increase INR → Increased risk of toxicity

Side-effects	• Common
	  – Antibiotic-associated diarrhoea
	  – Hypersensitivity reactions
	• Frequency not known:
	  – CNS toxicity
	  – False positive urinary glucose
		→ Not an allergy, but the drug's normal mode of action

Patient counselling	• **Complete antibiotic course:** failure to complete course may result in antibiotic resistance, making infections by the pathogen harder to treat in the future. • **Take before food:** some penicillins, such as flucloxacillin and phenoxymethylpenicillin, should be taken on an empty stomach. Patients should be advised to read the instruction leaflet with their medication for further instructions on use. • **Angioedema/allergic reaction:** if swelling of the face, eyes, lips or tongue develops or if breathing difficulties occur, call an ambulance. • **Important drug interactions:** some penicillins may increase your INR if taking warfarin so it might be necessary to get INR checked more regularly during antibiotic course.	→ If you miss a dose, take it as soon as you remember. Do not take two doses together.

Cephalosporins		
Examples	• 1st generation: cefalexin, cefradine, cefadroxil • 2nd generation: cefuroxime, cefaclor • 3rd generation: cefotaxime, ceftazidime, ceftriaxone	→ Start with cef-
Mode of action	• Inhibit cross-linking of peptide chains in the peptidoglycan bacterial cell wall, resulting in lysis of the weakened bacterial cell wall and cell death	→ Broad spectrum: effective in treating Gram +ve and Gram –ve bacteria, depending on indication → **Avoid over-prescribing of antibiotics (e.g. prescribing antibiotics when not indicated)** → **The rise of antibiotic-resistant bacteria is a serious challenge worldwide**
Routes of delivery	• PO, IV, IM	
Indications	• Septicaemia • Pneumonia • Peritonitis • Biliary tract infections • UTI • CNS infections (ceftriaxone and cefuroxime)	→ This indication is crucial to note as many other types of antibiotics do not cross the blood–brain barrier, thus they are not effective in CNS infections
Cautions and contraindications	• Contraindicated in patients with hypersensitivity reaction to penicillin (p. 104) • Use with caution in those at high risk of *C. difficile* infection and in renal impairment	
Interactions	• Aminoglycosides	→ Increased risk of nephrotoxicity
Monitoring	• Monitor WCC and CRP, review patient's clinical state	→ To look for signs of improvement and symptom resolution
Side-effects	• GI upset, diarrhoea, nausea and vomiting • Cholestatic jaundice (ceftriaxone) • Stevens–Johnson syndrome and toxic epidermal necrolysis • Please note that use of cephalosporins may result in false positive test results, such as false positive urinary glucose (if testing for reducing substances) and false positive Coombs' test	→ GI side-effects may be reduced by taking drug with food
Patient counselling	• ***Angioedema/allergic reaction:***	→ If swelling of the face, eyes, lips or tongue develops or if breathing difficulties occur, call an ambulance.

Carbapenems

Examples	• Meropenem, imipenem, ertapenem	→ End in -penem
Mode of action	• Inhibit cross-linking of peptide chains in the peptidoglycan bacterial cell wall, resulting in lysis of the weakened bacterial cell wall	→ Broad spectrum: effective in treating Gram +ve and Gram –ve bacteria, depending on indication → **Avoid over-prescribing of antibiotics (e.g. prescribing antibiotics when not indicated)** → **The rise of antibiotic-resistant bacteria is a serious challenge worldwide**
Route of delivery	• PO, IV	
Indications	• Severe hospital-acquired infections • Polymicrobial infections	
Cautions and contraindications	• Contraindicated in patients with hypersensitivity reaction to penicillin	
Monitoring	• Monitor WCC and CRP, review patient's clinical state	→ To look for signs of improvement
Interactions	• Sodium valproate	→ Reduced plasma concentration of sodium valproate

Side-effects	• Common or very common:
	  – GI disturbances, e.g. diarrhoea, nausea, vomiting
	  – Headache
	  – Mild skin reactions
	  – Pruritus
	  – Disturbances in LFTs	

Patient counselling	• ***Complete antibiotic course:*** • ***Do not take if allergic to penicillin:***	→ Failure to complete course may result in antibiotic resistance, making infections by the pathogen harder to treat in the future. → Ensure that patient is aware that they must avoid carbapenems if they are penicillin-allergic due to cross-sensitivity and that they should let healthcare professionals know about any drug allergies if having medical treatment.

Macrolides

Examples	• Clarithromycin, erythromycin, azithromycin	➤ End in -mycin ➤ Note that not all drugs that end in -mycin are macrolides, e.g. neomycin and tobramycin
Mode of action	• Inhibit bacterial synthesis by reversibly binding to the 50s subunit on the ribosome, preventing elongation of the bacterial protein chain	➤ Broad spectrum: effective in treating Gram positive and some Gram negative bacteria ➤ Alternative to penicillin in penicillin-allergic patients ➤ **Avoid over-prescribing of antibiotics (e.g. prescribing antibiotics when not indicated)** ➤ **The rise of antibiotic-resistant bacteria is a serious challenge worldwide**
Routes of delivery	• PO, IV	
Indications	• Respiratory tract infections • Mild–moderate soft tissue infections, e.g. cellulitis • As part of *H. pylori* eradication therapy (clarithromycin) • *Chlamydia trachomatis* • Acne rosacea (erythromycin) • Lyme disease	
Cautions and contraindications	• Patients who are prone to QT prolongation • Myasthenia gravis	➤ QT prolongation is a serious side-effect of this drug ➤ Condition can be exacerbated by macrolide use
Interactions	Please note that azithromycin does not inhibit cytochrome P450 and thus it is involved in very few drug interactions. Below is a list of the most common drug interactions with macrolides, some of which may not apply to azithromycin. • Warfarin • Statins • Carbamazepine • Theophylline and colchicine • Antipsychotics • Quinolones	 ➤ Increased anticoagulant effect and increased INR ➤ Increased risk of rhabdomyolysis (can be fatal) ➤ Increased serum carbamazepine levels due to CYP450 inhibition, which may result in toxicity ➤ Increased risk of toxicity ➤ Increased risk of arrhythmias ➤ Increased risk of QT prolongation and lowers seizure threshold
Monitoring	• Consider obtaining a baseline ECG • Macrolides can cause QT interval prolongation, hence ECGs can be considered if cardiac symptoms develop • Monitor INR closely in patients who take warfarin during treatment with a macrolide	➤ To exclude cardiac abnormalities that would increase patient's risk of developing QT prolongation ➤ To detect QT prolongation

Side-effects	• Common or very common:
	  – GI disturbances, e.g. abdominal pain, diarrhoea, nausea, vomiting
	• Uncommon or frequency not known:
	  – QT interval prolongation
	  – Hepatotoxicity
	  – Stevens–Johnson syndrome, toxic epidermal necrolysis
	  – Pancreatitis (rare)
	  – Cholestatic jaundice
	  – Hearing loss, generally reversible
		→ GI side-effects can be reduced by giving smaller doses in mild infections
		
		→ Can occur after large doses of macrolides, typically azithromycin

Patient counselling	• ***Complete antibiotic course:*** • ***Signs to watch out for:***	→ Failure to complete course may result in antibiotic resistance, making infections by the pathogen harder to treat in the future. → Inform a doctor if the following symptoms develop: severe abdominal pain, yellow discoloration of the skin or eyes, darkened urine, pale stools, or unusual tiredness.

Aminoglycosides

Examples	• Gentamicin, amikacin, neomycin, tobramycin	
Mode of action	• Inhibit bacterial synthesis by irreversibly binding to the 30s subunit on the ribosome, preventing elongation of the bacterial protein chain	→ Narrow spectrum: not effective against anaerobes. Effective against Gram +ve bacteria and some Gram –ve bacteria → **Avoid over-prescribing of antibiotics (e.g. prescribing antibiotics when not indicated)** → **The rise of antibiotic-resistant bacteria is a serious challenge worldwide**
Route of delivery	• IV, IM, topical (e.g. eye/ear drops)	→ Aminoglycosides are not well-absorbed in the gut → Avoid parenteral treatment for more than 7 days
Indications	• Meningitis • Septicaemia • Hospital-acquired pneumonia • Biliary tract infections • Acute pyelonephritis and prostatitis • Endocarditis • *Pseudomonas aeruginosa* infections	
Cautions and contraindications	• Severe renal impairment or renal failure • Myasthenia gravis • Intra-aural use not recommended in patients with patent grommets *in situ* • Avoid in 2nd and 3rd trimesters of pregnancy due to risk of causing auditory or vestibular nerve damage in infant	→ Aminoglycosides undergo renal excretion → Aminoglycosides are known to impair neuromuscular transmission
Monitoring	• Check renal function at baseline and during review appointments as per local guidelines • Serum aminoglycoside levels should be monitored as per local protocols	→ Avoids excessive and sub-therapeutic treatment → Target serum gentamicin levels: 5–12 mg/L at peak, <2 mg/L trough
Interactions	• Loop diuretics and vancomycin • NSAIDs, cephalosporins, ciclosporins, aciclovir, cisplatin, trimethoprim • Digoxin	→ Increased risk of ototoxicity → Increased risk of nephrotoxicity → Potential increase in serum digoxin concentration

Side-effects	• Rare or frequency not known:
	  – Antibiotic-associated colitis
	  – Electrolyte disturbances
	  – Hypocalcaemia
	  – Hypokalaemia
	  – Hypomagnesaemia
	  – Nausea	

Side-effects – **cont'd**	– Peripheral neuropathy – Nephrotoxicity – Ototoxicity – Neurotoxicity	
Patient counselling	• **_Complete antibiotic course:_** • **_Report problems with hearing or balance and stop drug:_**	→ Failure to complete course may result in antibiotic resistance, making infections by the pathogen harder to treat in the future. → May cause ototoxicity, hence patients should be advised to stop taking drug if hearing loss, tinnitus or problems with balance develop and to inform their doctor about these changes.

Glycopeptide antibiotics		
Examples	• Vancomycin, teicoplanin	
Mode of action	• Prevent elongation of peptide chain by inhibiting incorporation of NAMA and NAG subunits into chain	→ Narrow spectrum: effective against aerobic and anaerobic Gram +ve bacteria → **Avoid over-prescribing of antibiotics (e.g. prescribing antibiotics when not indicated)** → **The rise of antibiotic-resistant bacteria is a serious challenge worldwide**
Routes of delivery	• PO, IV **Note:** Vancomycin and teicoplanin should not be given orally in systemic infections as they are not well-absorbed	→ Slow administration IV is necessary to avoid anaphylactoid reactions or red man syndrome
Indications	• Infections by Gram +ve pathogens • *C. difficile* colitis • Endocarditis • Surgical prophylaxis when high risk for methicillin-resistant *S. aureus* (MRSA)	→ Can be given before and after the operation
Cautions and contraindications	• Avoid in patients with hearing loss • Dose should be reduced in renal impairment	
Interactions	• Vancomycin: loop diuretics, ciclosporin, tacrolimus, aminoglycosides • Teicoplanin: monitor renal and auditory function if prolonged administration and other nephrotoxic or neurotoxic drugs administered	→ Increased risk of nephrotoxicity
Monitoring	• Baseline U+Es and regular monitoring of renal function • Target vancomycin levels should be 5–15 mg/L trough or up to 20 mg/L in severe infections	→ To monitor signs of renal impairment

Side-effects	• Common:
	  – Ototoxicity (uncommon for teicoplanin, only if IV with vancomycin)
	  – Nephrotoxicity
	  – Pruritus
	  – Rash
	• Frequency not known:
	  – Red man syndrome (normally associated with rapid IV infusion rates)	

Patient counselling	• *Complete antibiotic course:* • *Ototoxicity:*	→ Failure to complete course may result in antibiotic resistance, making infections by the pathogen harder to treat in the future. → Advise patient to stop taking drug and contact their doctor if they develop hearing loss.

Tetracyclines

Examples	• Doxycycline, tigecycline, tetracycline	➤ End in -cycline
Mode of action	• Bind to the 30S ribosomal subunit to prevent tRNA binding, which inhibits bacterial protein synthesis	➤ Broad spectrum: effective against Gram +ve and –ve bacteria ➤ **Avoid over-prescribing of antibiotics (e.g. prescribing antibiotics when not indicated)** ➤ **The rise of antibiotic-resistant bacteria is a serious challenge worldwide**
Route of delivery	• PO, IV	
Indications	• Acute exacerbation of COPD • Intra-abdominal sepsis • Acne • Malaria	
Cautions and contraindications	• Contraindicated in children under 12, pregnant or breastfeeding women • Avoid in renal and hepatic impairment	➤ Tetracyclines interfere with calcium metabolism
Monitoring	• Monitor WCC and CRP, review patient's clinical state	➤ To look for signs of improvement
Interactions	• Warfarin • Antacids and milk	➤ Increased anticoagulant effect ➤ Reduced tetracycline absorption

Side-effects	• Rare or frequency not known:
	  – GI disturbances e.g. dysphagia, oesophageal irritation, nausea, vomiting, diarrhoea
	  – Tooth staining
	  – Hepatotoxicity
	  – Teratogenicity
	  – Antibiotic-associated colitis
	  – Headache
	  – Visual disturbances
	  – Benign intracranial hypertension
	  – Bulging fontanelles in infants
		➤ Causes skeletal development problems and stained teeth

Patient counselling	• *Complete antibiotic course:* • *Stained teeth:* • *Milk and antacids:*	➤ Failure to complete course may result in antibiotic resistance, making infections by the pathogen harder to treat in the future. ➤ Inform patient that drug may cause dental staining and its use should be avoided in children and pregnant or breastfeeding women. ➤ Inform patient not to take tetracyclines at the same time as taking antacids or drinking milk.

Quinolones		
Examples	• Ciprofloxacin, levofloxacin, ofloxacin	→ End in -floxacin
Mode of action	• Inhibit bacterial synthesis at an early stage by preventing supercoiling of the DNA double helix	→ Narrow spectrum: effective against Gram –ve bacteria and some Gram +ve bacteria → **Avoid over-prescribing of antibiotics (e.g. prescribing antibiotics when not indicated)** → **The rise of antibiotic-resistant bacteria is a serious challenge worldwide**
Routes of delivery	• PO, IV, topical including eye/ear drops	
Indications	• UTIs and prostatitis • Respiratory tract infections • GI infections • Ear infections	

Cautions and contraindications	• Contraindicated in:
	  – Children and adolescents
	  – Epilepsy and patients at high risk of seizures
	  – Patients with a history of tendon disorders related to quinolone use
	• Dose should be reduced in renal impairment
		→ Due to risk of causing arthropathy
		
		→ Advise patient to maintain sufficient fluid intake

Interactions	• Warfarin • NSAIDs • Antacids	→ Increased anticoagulant effect and increased INR → Increased risk of convulsions → Interfere with absorption of quinolones
Monitoring	• Monitor WCC and CRP, and review patient's clinical state	→ To look for signs of improvement

Side-effects	• Common:
	  – GI disturbances, headache, dizziness
	  – Night-time vision impairment
	• Less common:
	  – Rashes
	  – Tendon damage or rupture
	  – Arthropathy
	• Rare:
	  – Convulsions
		→ Increased risk in patients over 60 or taking corticosteroids
		
		→ Can cause seizures in patients with or without epilepsy

Patient counselling	• *Complete antibiotic course:* • *How to take*:	→ Failure to complete course may result in antibiotic resistance, making infections by the pathogen harder to treat in the future. → Maintain adequate fluid intake and do not take antacids at the same time as taking drug.

Patient counselling – cont'd	• **Risk of convulsions:**	→ Inform patients about the risk of convulsions and encourage the patient to inform those close to them about this risk, as other people may be required to seek medical help if the patient were to have a seizure.
	• **Tendon problems:**	→ It would be useful to inform patients about the risk of tendon damage or rupture, particularly those who are heavily involved with sports. Patients should stop taking quinolones immediately if signs of tendinitis develop. Patients over the age of 60 are more prone to tendon damage as well as those who take steroids concomitantly (BNF 2017).
	• **Driving:**	→ Quinolone use may impair the performance of normal activities such as driving.

Metronidazole

Examples	• Metronidazole	
Mode of action	• Binds to the DNA of specific pathogens, e.g. anaerobes and protozoa, resulting in cell death	➤ Narrow spectrum: effective against anaerobes and protozoa
Route of delivery	• PO, IV, PR	➤ Metronidazole is not well-absorbed orally, hence it should only be prescribed orally for mild infections
Indications	• Intra-abdominal sepsis • As part of *H. pylori* eradication therapy • Infection by *C. difficile* and other anaerobes • Protozoal infections • Dental infections	
Cautions and contraindications	• Use with caution in pregnant or breastfeeding women • Reduce dose in hepatic impairment • Avoid exposure to strong sunlight or UV light during topical use	➤ Monitor LFTs during treatment in hepatic impairment
Monitoring	• Monitor WCC and CRP, review patient's clinical state • If treatment exceeds 10 days, check LFTs for hepatotoxicity and FBC for blood dyscrasias	➤ To look for signs of improvement ➤ Long treatments with metronidazole are not advisable due to the risk of hepatotoxicity, blood dyscrasias and of developing peripheral neuropathy
Interactions	• Alcohol (causes disulfiram-like reaction) • Warfarin • Clozapine • Acitretin	➤ Can induce profuse vomiting when alcohol is consumed ➤ Increased anticoagulant effect ➤ Increased risk of agranulocytosis ➤ Increased risk of hepatotoxicity

Side-effects	• Very rare or frequency not known:
	  – Arthralgia
	  – Ataxia
	  – Dizziness
	  – Headache
	  – Blood dyscrasias
	  – Hepatitis and pancreatitis
	  – Metallic taste in mouth
	  – Peripheral neuropathy
	  – Dark urine	

Patient counselling	• ***Complete antibiotic course:*** • ***Reacts with alcohol:***	➤ Failure to complete course may result in antibiotic resistance, making infections by the pathogen harder to treat in the future. ➤ May cause vomiting, headache and dizziness when alcohol is consumed whilst taking drug, hence it is advisable to avoid alcohol whilst taking metronidazole and for 48 hours after stopping drug.

Nitrofurantoin

Examples	• Nitrofurantoin	
Mode of action	• Believed to inhibit enzymes involved in cell wall synthesis and bacterial carbohydrate metabolism	→ Narrow spectrum: not effective against all pathogens that cause UTIs, e.g. *Proteus* and *Pseudomonas* spp.
Routes of delivery	• PO, IV	
Indications	• Urinary tract infections	
Cautions and contraindications	• Contraindicated in acute porphyria, G6PD deficiencies, infants <3 months old • Avoid in at-term pregnancies and in breastfeeding • Use with caution in anaemia, B12 and folate deficiency, pulmonary disease, renal or hepatic impairment and in conditions associated with peripheral neuropathy	→ Teratogenic: may cause neonatal haemolysis
Interactions	• Oral magnesium salts	→ Reduced absorption of nitrofurantoin
Monitoring	• Monitor FBC during long-term treatment • Monitor lung function in long-term use	→ To detect and treat any blood disorders that occur → Stop nitrofurantoin if deterioration in lung function occurs

Side-effects	• Rare or frequency not known:
	  – Agranulocytosis
	  – Aplastic anaemia
	  – Arthralgia
	  – Blood disorders
	  – Cholestatic jaundice
	  – Hepatitis and pancreatitis
	  – Thrombocytopenia
	  – Alopecia
	  – Pulmonary fibrosis
	  – Peripheral neuropathy
	  – Haemolytic anaemia
	  – Hyperkalaemia
	  – Hypersensitivity reactions	

Patient counselling	• ***Complete antibiotic course:*** • ***How to take:*** • ***Brown urine:***	→ Failure to complete course may result in antibiotic resistance, making infections by the pathogen harder to treat in the future. → If taken as tablets, nitrofurantoin should be taken with food and must be swallowed whole. → Warn patients that this antibiotic may cause their urine to turn brown in colour.

Trimethoprim

Examples	• Trimethoprim	
Mode of action	• Inhibit dihydrofolate reductase, an enzyme that converts dihydrofolic acid (DHF) to tetrahydrofolic acid (THF), disrupting the bacterial synthesis pathway	→ Broad spectrum: effective against both Gram +ve and Gram −ve bacteria → **Avoid over-prescribing of antibiotics (e.g. prescribing antibiotics when not indicated)** → **The rise of antibiotic-resistant bacteria is a serious challenge worldwide**
Route of delivery	• PO	
Indications	• Urinary tract infections • Acute and chronic bronchitis • *Pneumocystis jirovecii* pneumonia	
Cautions and contraindications	• Blood dyscrasias • Pregnancy in the first trimester	→ Trimethoprim is a folate antagonist
Interactions	• Warfarin • ACEi and angiotensin receptor antagonists • Amiodarone • Azathioprine, mercaptopurine, methotrexate • Diuretics, amphotericin, aciclovir	→ Increased anticoagulant effect → Increased risk of hyperkalaemia → Increased risk of arrhythmias → Increased risk of haematological toxicity → Increased risk of nephrotoxicity
Monitoring	• Monitor FBC during long-term treatment	→ To detect and treat any blood disorders that occur

Side-effects	• Rare:
	  – Anaphylaxis and allergic reactions
	  – Angioedema
	  – Erythema multiforme and toxic epidermal necrolysis
	  – Photosensitivity
	• Frequency not known:
	  – Aseptic meningitis
	  – Hyperkalaemia
	  – Reduction in haematopoiesis
	  – Nausea
	  – Rashes
	  – Uveitis, reported in adults	

Patient counselling	• **_Complete antibiotic course:_**	➤ Failure to complete course may result in antibiotic resistance, making infections by the pathogen harder to treat in the future.
	• **_Not for use in pregnancy:_**	➤ Trimethoprim should be avoided in pregnancy as it may cause fetal anomalies, hence it is not recommended in pregnant women.
	• **_When to seek help:_**	➤ The patient should contact a doctor if they notice bleeding, bruising, rashes, fevers or sore throats whilst on trimethoprim.

Triazole antifungals

Examples	• Fluconazole, itraconazole	➤ End in -conazole
Mode of action	• Inhibit fungal cytochrome P450 3A enzyme which converts lanosterol to ergosterol (key component of fungal cell membrane), hence fungal cell replication is prevented	➤ Variable spectrum: some are broad spectrum, others are only effective against specific pathogens
Routes of delivery	• PO, IV, topical	
Indications	• Fungal respiratory tract infections, e.g. aspergillosis • Candidiasis • Skin and nail infections • Prophylaxis against fungal infections in immunocompromised patients	
Cautions and contraindications	• Contraindicated in acute porphyrias and should be used with caution in QT interval prolongation • Avoid in liver disease • Avoid fluconazole in pregnancy and only use itraconazole in life-threatening conditions	➤ May cause hepatotoxicity ➤ Teratogenic: may cause multiple congenital anomalies with high doses long-term
Interactions	• CCBs • Warfarin • Sulphonylureas • Colchicine	➤ Negative inotrope, can precipitate heart failure ➤ Increased anticoagulant effect ➤ Increased sulphonylurea concentration in plasma ➤ Increased risk of colchicine toxicity, hence colchicine should be withheld while antifungal is being taken
Monitoring	• Baseline ECG	➤ To detect ECG changes in the future

Side-effects	• Common or very common:
	  – GI disturbances, e.g. abdominal pain, nausea, diarrhoea
	  – Dyspnoea
	  – Headache
	  – Hepatitis
	  – Hypokalaemia
	  – Rash
	• Uncommon:
	  – Oedema
	  – Constipation, dyspepsia, flatulence
	  – Dizziness
	  – Peripheral neuropathy and myalgia
	  – Menstrual disorder	

Patient counselling	• **Complete antibiotic course:**	→	Failure to complete course may result in antibiotic resistance, making infections by the pathogen harder to treat in the future.
	• **Use reliable contraception whilst taking drug:**	→	Advise female patients to use reliable contraception during treatment and until next period after cessation of treatment, due to drug teratogenicity.
	• **Beware of signs of liver dysfunction:**	→	Stop drug immediately and contact your doctor if you develop abdominal pain, anorexia, nausea, vomiting, dark urine or pale stools.

Antivirals		
Examples	• Aciclovir, valaciclovir, ganciclovir, famciclovir	➔ End in -ciclovir
Mode of action	• Prevent DNA replication by terminating nucleotide chains	➔ Narrow spectrum: effective against viruses
Route of delivery	• PO, IV, topical	
Indications	• Herpes simplex and herpes zoster • Varicella zoster • Cytomegalovirus (CMV) (ganciclovir only)	
Cautions and contraindications	• Use with caution in the elderly • Reduce dose in renal impairment and advise patient to maintain hydration	
Monitoring	• Look for clinical signs of improvement • Monitor renal function if elderly or having long-term treatment	
Interactions	• Theophylline • Methotrexate, cephalosporins, ciclosporin, tacrolimus, NSAIDs	➔ Increased plasma concentration of theophylline ➔ Increased risk of nephrotoxicity

Side-effects	• Common:
	  – GI disturbances
	  – Fatigue
	  – Rash
	  – Headache
	  – Photosensitivity
	• Rare:
	  – Tremors
	  – Fever
	  – Psychosis	

Patient counselling	• ***Complete antiviral course:*** failure to complete the course may result in lack of treatment of virus and infection may persist. • ***Hygiene rules:*** do not touch eyes after touching cold sores. • ***Drink plenty of fluids:*** it is important to maintain hydration to reduce risk of renal impairment due to antiviral drug.	➔ If used as skin cream or eye ointment, it is important to apply antiviral medication 5 times daily

Paracetamol

Examples	• Paracetamol (acetaminophen)	→ Safest analgesic drug
Mode of action	• Believed to centrally inhibit COX-3 and weakly inhibit COX-2. COX inhibition is associated with increased pain threshold and reduction in prostaglandins	→ Does not inhibit COX-1 so it does not cause peptic ulceration and renal impairment
Route of delivery	• PO, IV, PR • Effervescent tablets are available but have a high sodium content	→ Avoid IV route in those with a body weight <50 kg and those with risk factors for hepatotoxicity, due to increased risk of toxicity (BNF 2017) → Avoid effervescent tablets in hypernatraemia
Indications	• Mild to moderate pain • Pyrexia • Post-immunization pyrexia (unlicensed)	→ Strong analgesic and anti-pyretic effects but weak anti-inflammatory effects
Cautions and contraindications	• Hepatocellular insufficiency • Chronic alcohol intoxication • Malnutrition – use with caution in patients with a body weight <50 kg	
Monitoring	• Review pain severity or measure temperature • In suspected or known paracetamol overdose, paracetamol serum levels must be checked 4 hours after ingestion or as per local guidelines	→ Paracetamol can take up to 30 minutes to start working
Interactions	• CYP450 inducers e.g. phenytoin, carbamazepine	→ Increase rate of NAPQI production (see *N*-acetylcysteine, p. 144) and increased risk of paracetamol toxicity

Side-effects	• Rare:
	  – Malaise
	  – Skin reactions such as acute generalized exanthematous pustulosis, toxic epidermal necrosis (TEN) and Stevens–Johnson syndrome
	  – Flushing and tachycardia (IV use)
	• Frequency not known:
	  – Blood disorders such as thrombocytopenia, neutropenia and leukopenia
	  – Hypotension (IV use)
	• In overdose
	  – Hepatocellular necrosis and acute renal tubular necrosis
		• Mnemonic **COMA (paracetamol toxicity risk factors)**
		  Chronic alcohol abusers
		  On drugs that induce cytochrome P450
		  Malnourished individuals
		  Anorexic individuals

Patient counselling	• ***Stick to prescribed dose:*** do not exceed maximum dose if pain uncontrolled. Do not take more than one dose to make up for missed doses. • ***Over-the-counter drugs:*** check labels of over-the-counter drugs as some combination medications may contain paracetamol, e.g. co-codamol. • ***Overdose:*** seek medical help immediately if you suspect that you or someone you know has taken an overdose of paracetamol.	→ Consider using other modes of analgesia when maximum dose has been reached

Non-steroidal anti-inflammatory drugs (NSAIDs)

Examples	• Non-selective: ibuprofen, diclofenac, naproxen • Selective: parecoxib	→ Target inflammatory cells; less likely to cause GI effects
Mode of action	• Block production of prostaglandins from arachidonic acid by inhibiting COX-1 and COX-2	→ Prostaglandins are mediators of inflammation and pain
Routes of delivery	• PO, IV	
Indications	• Mild to moderate pain • Inflammatory pain, particularly musculoskeletal pain • NSAIDs can be useful in back pain and soft tissue disorders (BNF 2017)	→ Examples include dental pain and dysmenorrhoea → Used to be 1st line in rheumatoid arthritis
Cautions and contraindications	• Asthma • Active gastric ulceration or bleeding • NSAID hypersensitivity • Renal impairment • Severe heart failure and liver failure • Pregnancy and breastfeeding – avoid in 3rd trimester due to risk of premature closure of ductus arteriosus	• Mnemonic **NSAID (NSAID contraindications)** **N**ursing a baby (pregnancy and breastfeeding) **S**evere bleeding **A**sthma **I**ssues with renal function **D**rug allergy
Interactions	• Corticosteroids, aspirin • Anticoagulants, other NSAIDs, SSRIs, venlafaxine • Nephrotoxic drugs, e.g. aminoglycosides, ACEi, ARBs • Lithium	→ Increased risk of GI ulceration → Increased risk of GI bleeding → Increased risk of renal impairment → Increased risk of lithium toxicity and renal impairment
Monitoring	• U+Es before starting treatment	→ To check baseline renal function

Side-effects	• Frequency not known:
	  – Headaches – GI irritation, GI ulceration and GI bleeding
	  – Dizziness – Bronchospasm (if given to asthmatics)
	  – Nausea – Renal impairment (impaired renal blood flow)
	  – Diarrhoea
	• All NSAID use is associated with a small increased risk of thrombotic events regardless of patient's baseline cardiovascular risk factors or duration of NSAID treatment (BNF 2017)
		→ Advise patients to stop NSAID if dehydrated, to avoid further renal damage

Patient counselling	• *Reducing GI effects:* • *Allergic reaction:* • *Alcohol:*	→ Taking drug with food may help to minimize indigestion. In long-term NSAID use, a PPI should be taken to protect the gastric mucosa. → If swelling of the face, eyes, lips or tongue develops or if breathing difficulties occur, stop taking drug and call an ambulance immediately. → Alcohol increases the risk of GI bleeding, therefore it is not recommended for moderate drinkers to use NSAIDs, and those who exceed the recommended daily limits of alcohol should exercise greater caution (BNF 2017).

Codeine		
Examples	• Codeine phosphate, dihydrocodeine (weak opioids)	
Mode of action	• Simultaneously acts at the opioid receptors to cause euphoria and analgesia, and at the medulla to suppress the cough reflex	
Route of delivery	• PO, IM	➤ Available as slow release ➤ Not for IV administration – causes reaction similar to anaphylaxis
Indications	• Mild to moderate pain of acute or chronic nature • Diarrhoea • Cough suppression	➤ Most commonly used weak opioid for pain relief
Cautions and contraindications	• All opioids are contraindicated in respiratory depression, head injury, raised intracranial pressure and in patients at risk of paralytic ileus • Codeine is contraindicated in acute ulcerative colitis, antibiotic-associated colitis, in known ultra-rapid codeine metabolizers (see *Note* below) and in <18-year-olds who have undergone tonsillectomy or adenoidectomy to treat sleep apnoea • Codeine should be avoided in breastfeeding • Codeine should be avoided in renal and hepatic impairment **Note:** There is a variation in metabolism. Some patients are CYP2D6 ultra-rapid codeine metabolizers and are at high risk of opioid toxicity, whereas other patients are slow metabolizers.	➤ There have been reports of deaths following codeine use in this paediatric population due to respiratory depression. ➤ MHRA has recommended that codeine is only used to treat acute severe pain in >12-year-olds if other non-opioid analgesics have failed to control the child's pain (MHRA July 2013); further MHRA/CHM guidance has been issued warning against prescribing codeine as a cold and cough suppressant in children <12 (MHRA/CHM April 2015) ➤ See section on breastfeeding in *Patient counselling*, below ➤ Codeine is metabolized by the liver and excreted by the kidneys
Monitoring	• Review the pain control within hours of taking codeine in acute pain or schedule a timely review of pain control in patients with chronic pain	
Interactions	• Alcohol, sedatives, hypnotics, general anaesthetic agents	➤ Depress the central nervous system and increase risk of respiratory depression

Side-effects	• Common:
	  – Nausea and vomiting
	  – Constipation
	  – Respiratory depression
	  – Hypotension
	  – Paralytic ileus
	  – Provoked seizures by lowering seizure threshold
		Mnemonic **CODEINE (codeine side-effects)**
		COnstipation
		Depression (respiratory)
		Emesis
		Ileus
		Nausea
		Exacerbates seizure activity

Codeine – *cont'd*

| Patient counselling | • **Impairment of normal abilities:** codeine may affect your ability to drive or operate machinery due to sedative effects. Do not drive or operate machinery if you feel dizzy or drowsy after taking this medication. Driving at the start of opioid therapy, and following dose changes, is not recommended (BNF 2017).
• **Bowel obstruction:** excessive codeine use can cause mechanical and paralytic bowel obstruction, so patients should be warned to stop taking codeine if bloating or distension occur (Richards and Aronson, *Oxford Handbook of Practical Drug Therapy*, 2005, p. 665)
• **Breastfeeding:** it is preferable to avoid codeine since it enters the breast milk in small amounts.
• **Alcohol:** avoid alcohol whilst taking opioids due to the increased risk of respiratory depression, since both drugs depress the central nervous system. | → As the ability of mothers to metabolize codeine varies, use can result in opioid overdose in the infant |

Tramadol

Examples	• Tramadol (weak opioid)	
Mode of action	Tramadol has two functions: • Acts as an agonist for the opioid μ receptors • Inhibits serotonin and noradrenaline reuptake	→ 10% of morphine's potency → Produces feelings of euphoria, in addition to pain relief
Routes of delivery	• PO, IV, IM	
Indications	• Moderate to severe pain	→ Often prescribed to post-surgical patients
Cautions and contraindications	• All opioids are contraindicated in respiratory depression, head injury, raised intracranial pressure and in patients at risk of paralytic ileus • Tramadol is contraindicated in uncontrolled epilepsy and in acute intoxication with alcohol, hypnotics or other opioids • Consider reducing tramadol doses in renal and hepatic impairment	→ May lower seizure threshold
Monitoring	• Review the pain control within hours of patient taking tramadol in acute pain or schedule a timely review of pain control in patients with chronic pain	
Interactions	• SSRIs, MAOIs, lithium and St John's wort • Alcohol	→ Increased risk of serotonin syndrome → Increased risk of CNS depression
Side-effects	• Same as codeine (see p. 126), but causes less constipation and less respiratory depression than codeine	→ Useful in postoperative patients
Patient counselling	• *Impairment of normal abilities:* • *Alcohol use not recommended:*	→ Tramadol may affect ability to drive or operate machinery due to sedative effects. Do not drive or operate machinery if you feel dizzy or drowsy after taking this medication. Driving at the start of opioid therapy, and following dose changes, is not recommended (BNF 2017). → Avoid alcohol whilst taking opioids due to the increased risk of respiratory depression, since both drugs depress the central nervous system.

Morphine

Examples	• Morphine (strong opioid)	
Mode of action	• Full agonist for G-protein coupled receptors	➤ Stronger effect than codeine and tramadol
Route of delivery	• PO, IV, IM, S/C, PR, epidural or intrathecal • Via patient-controlled analgesia (PCA)	➤ PCA has lock-out mechanism in place to prevent accidental overdose
Indications	• Moderate to severe pain of acute or chronic nature • Palliative treatment	➤ Escalate pain relief based on the pain ladder before prescribing morphine ➤ To keep patients comfortable at the end of life
Cautions and contraindications	• All opioids are contraindicated in respiratory depression, head injury, raised intracranial pressure and in patients at risk of paralytic ileus • Morphine is contraindicated in acute abdomen, delayed gastric emptying, heart failure secondary to chronic lung disease and in phaeochromocytoma (BNF 2017)	
Monitoring	• Sedation scores can be used to monitor patient	➤ The reversal agent for opioid-induced respiratory and CNS depression is naloxone, see p. 145
Interactions	• CNS depressants: alcohol, sedatives, anaesthetic agents • MAOIs	➤ Increased risk of respiratory depression ➤ Enhanced effects of morphine

Side-effects	• Common or very common (list not exhaustive but most significant side-effects stated below; refer to latest BNF for complete list):
	  – Nausea and vomiting
	  – Constipation
	  – Urinary retention
	  – Itching (due to histamine release)
	  – Respiratory depression
	  – Hypotension
	  – Paralytic ileus
	  – Sedation
	• Frequency not known:
	  – Following long-term use, adrenal insufficiency, hyperalgesia and hypogonadism can occur
		Mnemonic **MORPHINE (morphine side-effects)**
		Myosis
		Out of it (sedation)
		Respiratory depression
		Paralytic ileus
		Hypotension
		Infrequent opening of bowels and bladder
		Nausea
		Emesis

| Patient counselling | • **Impairment of normal abilities:** morphine may affect ability to drive or operate machinery due to sedative effects. Do not drive or operate machinery if you feel dizzy or drowsy after taking this medication.
 • **Alcohol use not recommended:** avoid alcohol whilst taking opioids due to the increased risk of respiratory depression, since both drugs depress the central nervous system. | **OPIOID EQUIVALENCY:**
 10 mg morphine PO = 100 mg codeine PO
 10 mg morphine PO = 67 mg tramadol PO
 10 mg morphine PO = 6.6 mg oxycodone PO
 10 mg morphine PO = 5 mg morphine S/C
 10 mg morphine PO = 5 mg morphine IV
 10 mg morphine PO = 5 mg morphine IM
 45 mg morphine PO = 12 micrograms/hour fentanyl patch
 (12 micrograms is the lowest dose of fentanyl and doses should be titrated up by increments of 12–25 micrograms) |

Fentanyl		
Examples	• Fentanyl (strong opioid)	
Mode of action	• Acts as an agonist for the opioid μ receptor	→ Produces similar (but weaker) effects to morphine
Routes of delivery	• PO, IV, topical (patch, film, spray) **Note:** Fentanyl is not the only opioid that can be administered as a patch; buprenorphine patches exist and they are used 1 patch per week	→ Patches are normally changed every 72 hours → Fentanyl preparations for breakthrough pain are not interchangeable
Indications	• Severe chronic pain • Breakthrough pain	→ Titrate dose up in increments of 12–25 micrograms/hour
Cautions and contraindications	• Same as morphine, see p. 129 • Use with caution in patients with impaired consciousness or cerebral tumours (fentanyl can worsen CNS depression in these conditions) and in mucositis (oral absorption can be altered)	
Monitoring	• Monitor pain relief at least 24 hours after altering a dose, to allow analgesic effect to occur	
Interactions	• Triazole antifungals	→ Increased plasma concentration of fentanyl

Side-effects	• Common or very common:
	  – Application-site reactions
	
	  – Abdominal pain, nausea, GORD and appetite changes
	  – Dyspnoea and respiratory depression
	  – Drowsiness
	  – Hypertension
	• Uncommon:
	  – Amnesia, arthralgia, ileus
	• Rare:
	  – Hiccups
	• IV fentanyl can cause muscle rigidity which can be managed with neuromuscular relaxants; patients with fentanyl patches should be monitored for increased side-effects if fever present and they should avoid exposing patches to external heat, e.g. saunas and hot baths (BNF 2017)
		→ Patients with severe side-effects should be monitored for 24 hours after patch removal

Patient counselling	• ***How to apply patches:*** • ***Drowsiness and impairment of normal activities:***	→ Fentanyl patches should be applied to dry, hairless areas of skin and then removed and changed after 72 hours. It is advisable to avoid using the same area multiple times in a row. Avoid exposing patches to external heat, e.g. saunas and hot baths. → Be aware that fentanyl may cause drowsiness and impairment of normal abilities such as driving.

Local anaesthetics (LA)

Examples	• Lidocaine (also known as lignocaine), bupivacaine	
Mode of action	• Reversibly blocks Na⁺ channels to prevent neurotransmission	➤ Mechanism behind nerve block
	• Causes vasodilatation of arteries; however, addition of adrenaline to prolong anaesthetic effects may counteract this effect as it is a vasoconstrictor	➤ Beware of injecting LA mixed with adrenaline into organs with end-artery blood supply
Route of delivery	• Topical, IV, epidural	➤ Can be mixed with adrenaline ➤ For non-emergency indications, doses should be calculated using ideal body weight ➤ May be applied topically with occlusive dressing
Indications	• Local anaesthetic for procedures • Treatment and prevention of ventricular tachycardia (VT) and ventricular fibrillation (VF) post-MI **Note:** In addition to local anaesthesia, these agents can be used for surface and infiltration anaesthesia, nerve blocks and epidural blocks.	
Cautions and contraindications	• Contraindicated in severe myocardial depression, sinoatrial disorders and in AV block • Avoid lidocaine in pregnancy • Dose reduction should occur in low cardiac output states	➤ Can cause neonatal bradycardia and, following large doses, respiratory and CNS depression (Richards and Aronson, *Oxford Handbook of Practical Drug Therapy*, 2005, p. 678)
Monitoring	• Sensation can be tested by touching the area where the local anaesthetic has been used with the needle tip and asking patient if the area feels numb or sharp	➤ To determine whether the local anaesthetic agent has taken effect
Interactions	• Adrenaline	➤ Prolongs anaesthetic effect
Side-effects	• Common: – Bradycardia – Dizziness – Hypotension – Drowsiness – Confusion – Respiratory depression – Convulsions • Rare: – Cardiac arrest in overdose	➤ There is a reversal agent for local anaesthetic-induced cardiac arrest, which is lipid-soluble and absorbs the local anaesthetic molecules
Patient counselling	• ***Effect of local anaesthetic:***	➤ The local anaesthetic will cause temporary loss of sensation (numbness) to the affected area. The patient might feel some stinging but this should not hurt and if the patient feels pain at any time during the procedure, they should inform the healthcare professional performing the procedure.

Adrenaline		
Examples	• Adrenaline (epinephrine)	
Mode of action	• Alpha- and beta-adrenoceptor agonist	➤ Acts on both alpha and beta receptors and increases both heart rate and contractility (beta$_1$ effects); it can cause peripheral vasodilatation (a beta$_2$ effect) or vasoconstriction (an alpha effect) (BNF 2017)
Route of delivery	• IM, IV or via nebulizer (in croup)	➤ IV adrenaline should only be used in cardiac arrests and by individuals who are trained in its use; resuscitation equipment must be available
Indications	• Anaphylaxis • Cardiopulmonary resuscitation (CPR) • Bronchodilator in airway obstruction • Local vasoconstriction, e.g. to stop bleeding during endoscopy or mixed with local anaesthetic drugs	➤ This can be self-administered IM by the patient using auto-injector device ➤ Also suppresses mast cell release in inflammation
Cautions and contraindications	• No contraindications to anaphylaxis treatment or CPR • Use with caution in patients with IHD and other cardiovascular conditions, diabetes mellitus • Mixed with local anaesthetic: not to be used in organs with end-artery blood supply	➤ Examples include the nose, the external ear, the digits and genitalia (risk of tissue necrosis)
Monitoring	• Monitor vital signs during and after treatment	
Interactions	• Beta blockers • MAOIs	➤ Increased risk of hypertension ➤ Concurrent use may increase risk of hypertensive crisis

Side-effects	• Frequency not known:
	  – Cardiovascular: angina, myocardial infarction, palpitations, tachycardia, arrhythmias, hypertension, cold extremities, pallor
	  – Respiratory: dyspnoea, pulmonary oedema
	  – GI: nausea, anorexia, vomiting, hypersalivation
	  – Genitourinary: urinary retention, difficulty in micturition
	  – CNS: anxiety, restlessness, insomnia, tremor, sweating, psychosis, confusion, weakness, dizziness
	  – Endocrine: hyperglycaemia, metabolic acidosis, hypokalaemia
	  – Ophthalmic: angle-closure glaucoma, mydriasis
	  – Tissue necrosis	

| Patient counselling | • ***Educate patient to self-administer adrenaline IM:*** | → Demonstrate IM administration to patient and ensure that the patient knows how to use auto-injector device by asking patient to demonstrate this skill with an unfilled device. Provide written information to patient to take home after consultation. |
| | • ***Carry auto-injector device with you at all times:*** | → Advise patients with known allergies to carry an adrenaline injection device (e.g. EpiPen) with them at all times. It is important to check expiry dates for your auto-injector devices. |

Amiodarone

Examples	• Amiodarone	
Mode of action	• Blocks sodium, calcium and potassium channels • Blocks alpha- and beta-adrenergic receptors	→ Prolongs the cardiac action potential, slows the heart rate → Decreases heart rate and blood pressure
Routes of delivery	• IV, PO	→ Highly irritant to skin: if a patient requires repeated or continuous infusion of amiodarone, it is recommended to site a central venous catheter
Indications	• Cardiopulmonary resuscitation • Rhythm control in AF • Atrial flutter and tachyarrhythmias in Wolff–Parkinson–White syndrome (WPW)	→ Non-shockable rhythms or following 3 unsuccessful DC shocks (Resuscitation Council UK, 2015)
Cautions and contraindications	• Contraindicated in sinus bradycardia, sinoatrial heart block, thyroid dysfunction and iodine sensitivity • Use with caution in hypokalaemia, severe bradycardia, heart failure and in the elderly	
Interactions	• Warfarin • Digoxin • Beta blockers, CCBs • Lithium, TCAs • Grapefruit juice Note that amiodarone has a long half-life and drug interactions may occur for several weeks (or even months) after treatment cessation	→ Increased anticoagulant effect → Increased plasma concentration of digoxin – dose needs to be adjusted → Increased risk of bradycardia and heart block → Increased risk of ventricular arrhythmias → Grapefruit juice increases exposure to amiodarone – manufacturer advises to avoid (BNF, 2017)
Monitoring	• Baseline CXR before starting treatment • Baseline TFTs and LFTs before starting treatment and re-checked every 6 months	→ Due to risk of pulmonary fibrosis → Due to risk of thyroid disease and hepatotoxicity

Side-effects	• Common or very common:
	  – Bradycardia
	  – Thyroid dysfunction
	  – Pulmonary fibrosis
	  – Photosensitivity
	  – Corneal microdeposits, sometimes causing night glare
	  – Peripheral neuropathy
	  – Jaundice
	  – Hepatotoxicity
	  – Vomiting
	  – Tremor
	  – Taste disturbances
	  – May raise serum transaminases
		→ Can cause hypo- or hyperthyroidism

Side-effects – **cont'd**	• Uncommon:
	   – Peripheral neuropathy and myopathy (reversible)
	   – Conduction disturbances
	   – Worsening arrhythmias
	• Very rare:
	   – Alopecia
	   – Optic neuritis
		→ Stop amiodarone and consider an alternative
		
		→ Amiodarone damages the optic nerve and it must be stopped in optic neuritis as blindness can occur

Patient counselling	• *Serious adverse effects:* • *Photosensitivity:* • *Optic neuritis:*	→ Inform the patient of the adverse effects and emphasize the importance of complying with monitoring, e.g. attending appointments for blood tests. → Advise patient to protect skin from direct sunlight. → Counsel patient about the signs and symptoms of optic neuritis and warn them that amiodarone must be stopped immediately as blindness can occur.

Adenosine

Examples	• Adenosine	
Mode of action	• Binds to G-protein coupled receptors	➤ Slows heart rate
Routes of delivery	• IV	➤ Lower doses should be prescribed if administered via central line compared to peripheral line ➤ Repeated doses may need to be given due to $t_{1/2}$ of <10 seconds.
Indications	• Supraventricular tachycardia (SVT)	➤ 1st line drug for diagnosis and therapeutic relief ➤ If true SVT, adenosine should revert rhythm to sinus rhythm
Cautions and contraindications	• Contraindicated in asthma, COPD, decompensated heart failure, cardiac transplant patients, 3rd degree AV block, sick sinus syndrome and severe hypotension • Use with caution in AF and atrial flutter with accessory pathways, 1st degree AV block, bundle branch block, autonomic dysfunction, recent MI, severe heart failure, stenotic and valvular heart disease, pericarditis and QT interval prolongation	
Monitoring	• Cardiac monitoring is compulsory during administration of adenosine and facilities for resuscitation should be available	➤ To check for return of sinus rhythm
Interactions	• Theophylline, aminophylline, caffeine	➤ Compete with adenosine for binding to G-protein coupled receptors
Side-effects	Note that IV injection with adenosine can be painful for the patient! • Common or very common: 　– Angina, bradycardia or asystole 　– Dyspnoea, bronchospasm 　– Flushing, headache • Uncommon: 　– Blurred vision 　– Hyperventilation 　– Metallic taste 　– Sweating 　– Palpitations 　– Weakness • Very rare: 　– Bronchospasm 　– Injection-site reactions 　– Transient worsening of intracranial hypertension	➤ Adenosine has a $t_{1/2}$ of <10 seconds, so doses may need to be repeated

Side-effects – **cont'd**	• Frequency not known:
	  – Cardiac arrest
	  – Convulsions
	  – Hypotension
	  – Respiratory failure
	  – Vomiting	

Patient counselling	• *Painful injection:*	→ Warn patient in advance about the severe pain associated with adenosine administration and that it can cause dyspnoea, bronchospasm and bradycardia.

Atropine

Examples	• Atropine	
Mode of action	• Muscarinic acetylcholine antagonist that blocks vagal input to SA and AV nodes	→ Counteracts bradycardia by increasing cardiac conduction → Can reverse AV block and restore normal sinus rhythm → This effect is short-lived and temporary due to short $t_{1/2}$
Routes of delivery	• PO, IV, IM	→ Pre-filled syringes exist; however, IV atropine should only be administered by individuals trained in its use
Indications	• Bradycardia • Organophosphorus poisoning • GI smooth muscle spasm	
Cautions and contraindications	• Contraindicated in myasthenia gravis, narrow-angle glaucoma, pyloric stenosis and prostatic hypertrophy • Avoid in children, elderly patients and those with Down syndrome • Use with caution in cardiovascular disease, arrhythmias, autonomic neuropathy, individuals susceptible to angle-closure glaucoma and hypertension	→ Reduced detrusor muscle activity results in urinary retention
Interactions	• SSRIs, TCAs, haloperidol, other antimuscarinic agents, codeine • Levodopa	→ Increased antimuscarinic side-effects of atropine → Reduced absorption of atropine
Monitoring	• Close monitoring of vital signs and ECG in emergency use of atropine during bradycardia	→ The effects of atropine wear off quickly due to its short half-life, hence close monitoring of the patient is required

Side-effects	• Common or very common:
	  – Increased heart rate (intended in bradycardia)
	  – Reduction in secretions, e.g. dry mouth
	  – Urinary retention
	  – Dilated pupils resulting in blurred vision
	  – Constipation
		→ Repeated doses may be required due to short $t_{1/2}$

Patient counselling	• *As drug is given in emergency situations, such as life-threatening bradycardia, sometimes patient counselling will not be possible; however, the prescriber should be aware of associated adverse effects and be able to explain them to the patient. The need for repeated doses, if required, should be explained to patients who are conscious during administration.* • ***Starting patients on atropine in the non-emergency setting:***	→ Inform patients that atropine tablets should be swallowed whole and warn patients about the antimuscarinic side-effects e.g. blurred vision, dry mouth, urinary retention and constipation.

Calcium gluconate

Examples	• Calcium gluconate	
Mode of action	• Raises the threshold potential for transmission of cardiac action potential by restoring the gap between resting membrane potential and threshold potential (this gap has been reduced in hyperkalaemia which increases cardiac excitability) **Note:** Calcium gluconate does not affect serum potassium levels; therefore patients with hyperkalaemia should receive insulin as per protocol. Salbutamol can be administered to help move K⁺ out of cells.	→ Stabilizes myocardium and prevents arrhythmias
Route of delivery	• IV	→ Administered into large vein over 5–10 min
Indications	• Hyperkalaemia • Severe acute hypocalcaemia or hypocalcaemic tetany	→ As per local guidelines for hyperkalaemia management
Cautions and contraindications	• Contraindicated in hypercalcaemia • Guidance from the MHRA states that repeated or prolonged administration of calcium gluconate injection packages in 10 ml glass containers in <18-year-olds and patients with renal impairment is contraindicated due to the risk of aluminium accumulation. It recommends use of calcium gluconate stored in plastic containers in these groups (BNF 2017) • Avoid in patients taking digoxin unless ECG shows changes in keeping with hyperkalaemia	
Monitoring	• Check ECG before and after treatment to look for resolution of tall tented T waves and flattened P waves, i.e. return to a normal ECG	→ To check for stabilization of the heart rhythm
Interactions	• Digoxin • Thiazide diuretics, indapamide • Levothyroxine, alendronic acid, ibandronic acid, risedronate sodium	→ Increased risk of digoxin toxicity → Increased risk of hypercalcaemia → Oral calcium gluconate can reduce absorption of these drugs. Consult patient information leaflets or speak to a pharmacist for further information regarding the appropriate time gap between taking the two medications
Side-effects	• If administered too fast: cardiovascular collapse • If administered subcutaneously: local tissue damage	
Patient counselling	• ***Explain need for treatment:***	→ Explain that the patient is having calcium gluconate, other drugs (insulin and salbutamol) and intravenous fluids in order to treat hyperkalaemia, which is a medical emergency, and that monitoring (blood tests and repeat ECGs) will be required.

Glucagon		
Examples	• Glucagon	
Mode of action	• Beta-2 agonist • Glucagon is a hormone produced by alpha cells in the islet of Langerhans in the pancreas • It mobilizes glycogen from the liver to be converted into glucose	→ Conversion of glycogen to glucose increases glucose levels in the body
Routes of delivery	• IM, IV, S/C	→ If not effective in hypoglycaemia, IV glucose should be administered
Indications	• Hypoglycaemia • Beta blocker overdose	→ Glucagon is not effective in chronic hypoglycaemia
Cautions and contraindications	• Phaeochromocytoma • Use with caution in glucagonoma, insulinoma, starvation and adrenal insufficiency • If glucagon is used to treat growth hormone secretion disorders in children, delayed hypoglycaemia may occur and it is essential to ensure that the child has a meal before discharge (BNF 2017)	
Interactions	• Warfarin	→ Increased anticoagulant effect
Monitoring	• In hypoglycaemia: monitor patient's blood glucose frequently • In beta blocker overdose: monitor patient's vital signs and treat symptomatically	→ To detect clinical benefit of glucagon
Side-effects	• Nausea and vomiting • Abdominal pain • Hypokalaemia • Hypotension	
Patient counselling	• ***Counselling on prevention and management of hypoglycaemia:***	→ Hypoglycaemia advice needs to be reinforced, see *Chapter 6*. Provide written advice in addition to verbal information about prevention and treatment of hypoglycaemia, and document this.

Phenytoin

Examples	• Phenytoin	
Mode of action	• Blocks voltage-gated Na⁺ channels	→ Stabilizes the presynaptic membrane and reduces seizure activity
Route of delivery	• IV	→ Prescribed by weight
Indications	• Status epilepticus • Epilepsy with the exception of absence seizures	
Cautions and contraindications	• Contraindicated in acute porphyrias and IV use • Contraindicated in sinus bradycardia, sinoatrial block, 2nd and 3rd degree heart block and Stokes–Adams syndrome • Caution in enteral feeding, which must be stopped 2 hours before and after phenytoin dose • Caution with IV use in heart failure, hypotension, respiratory depression and note that injection solutions are alkaline and may irritate tissues • Consider vitamin D supplementation in patients with long-term immobilization and patients with inadequate exposure to sun or calcium in their diet	
Monitoring	• Phenytoin has a narrow therapeutic index, thus monitoring of plasma phenytoin concentration must occur • Target phenytoin levels should be 8–15 mg/L	→ Follow local guidelines regarding plasma phenytoin concentration
Interactions	• Oral contraceptive pill • Theophylline and cimetidine • Amiodarone	→ Reduced contraceptive effect; consider alternative method of contraception if taking phenytoin → Reduced plasma concentration of phenytoin → Increased plasma concentration of phenytoin

Side-effects	• Common or very common:
	  – Skin changes: acne, hirsutism, hyperplasia of gums, yellow-brown discoloration
	  – CNS: nystagmus, vertigo, ataxia, tremor and headaches, paraesthesia, insomnia
	  – GI: nausea, anorexia, vomiting
	  – MSK: osteomalacia
	
	• Phenytoin is known to be teratogenic
	• Causes CYP450 inhibition (depends on effect on concurrent drugs)
		• Mnemonic **PHENYTOIN (phenytoin side-effects)**
		P450 inhibition
		Hirsutism
		Enlarged gums
		Nystagmus
		Yellow-brown discoloration of skin
		Teratogenicity
		Osteomalacia
		Interferes with folate metabolism
		Neuropathy

Patient counselling	• *When drug is given in status epilepticus, patient counselling will be not be possible; however, the prescriber should be aware of adverse effects and be able to explain them if needed.* • ***Teratogenicity:*** • ***Signs of blood disorders:***	→ Long-term use of phenytoin is associated with congenital abnormalities, hence it should be avoided in pregnant women. → Patient should contact a doctor if they develop a fever, rash, mouth ulcer, bleeding or bruising.

N-acetylcysteine (NAC)

Examples	• *N*-acetylcysteine (NAC)	
Mode of action	• Increases body's supply of glutathione, which conjugates with NAPQI (*N*-acetyl-*p*-benzoquinone imine) • NAPQI is produced as a by-product of paracetamol metabolism and in its free form, NAPQI causes liver damage	→ NAC is most effective when administered within 8 hours of ingestion of paracetamol overdose
Routes of delivery	• IV, PO	
Indications	• Paracetamol overdose • Prophylaxis of renal injury following contrast nephropathy • Mucolysis (respiratory secretions)	
Contraindications	• No absolute contraindications exist • Caution with IV use in atopy and in asthma, but do not delay treatment • Caution with oral use in children with asthma or children with a history of peptic ulceration	→ NAC is used in life-threatening paracetamol overdose
Interactions	• Frequency not known: – NAC may increase the INR and prothrombin time, thus caution should be exercised in patients taking warfarin	
Monitoring	• Monitor LFTs, coagulation screen before and after treatment with NAC	
Side-effects	• Hypersensitivity-like reactions (rare)	→ Reduce infusion rate or wait until reaction settles → Rashes can be treated with antihistamines → Shortness of breath can be treated with a beta-2 agonist
Patient counselling	• ***Explain treatment:***	→ Warn patient that the NAC infusion is run over many hours and that the patient will require blood tests before and after, for monitoring purposes.

Naloxone		
Examples	• Naloxone	
Mode of action	• Competes with opioid analgesics for binding to opioid receptors	→ Naloxone is short-acting, hence it might be necessary to repeat doses → The initial resuscitative dose is the dose that maintains ventilation for 15 minutes
Route of delivery	• IV, IM, S/C or continuous IV infusion	
Indications	• Opioid overdose • Postoperative respiratory depression • Neonatal respiratory depression following administration of opioid analgesia to mother during labour	→ Signs: reduced Glasgow Coma Score (GCS), low respiratory rate, pinpoint pupils
Contraindications	• Avoid in pregnancy • Caution in cardiac disease or use of cardiotoxic drugs, pain and physical dependence on opioids	
Monitoring	• Monitoring of vital signs, especially respiratory rate and oxygen saturations	→ Normally given in emergencies and it is essential the patient's airway is supported
Interactions	• No clinically significant interactions apart from interactions with opioids	

Side-effects	• Common or very common:
	  – Reversal of pain control
	  – Nausea
	  – Vomiting
	  – Dyspnoea
	  – Hypotension
	  – Dizziness
	  – Tachycardia
	  – Pulmonary oedema
	• Uncommon or rare:
	  – Agitation
	  – Arrhythmia
	  – Bradycardia
	  – Physical dependence
	  – Seizures
		• Mnemonic **NALOXONE (naloxone side-effects)**
		Nausea
		Agitation
		LOss of pain control
		e**X**citation (restlessness)
		Opioid dependence
		Neurological symptoms (fits)
		Elevated pulse rate

Patient counselling	• *As drug is given in emergency situations, such as respiratory depression, it is unlikely that patient counselling will be required; however, the prescriber should be aware of adverse effects, e.g. reversal of pain control, and be able to explain them if needed.*	

Benzodiazepine antagonists

Examples	• Flumazenil
Mode of action	• Compete with benzodiazepines for binding to GABA$_A$ receptors → Counteracts effects of benzodiazepine overdose by occupying receptors for binding
Routes of delivery	• IV
Indications	• Benzodiazepine overdose • Reversal of benzodiazepine-related sedation
Contraindications	• Contraindicated in status epilepticus and life-threatening conditions controlled by benzodiazepines • Avoid rapid injection following major surgery or in anxious patients • Breastfeeding should be avoided for 24 hours after taking drug • Caution in the elderly, those with physical dependence, history of panic disorders or receiving benzodiazepine treatment for epilepsy
Interactions	• TCAs
Monitoring	• Monitor patient's vital signs and neurological state during and after administration → To detect clinical benefit of drug

Side-effects	• Common or very common:
	  – Nausea and vomiting
	• Uncommon or frequency not known:
	  – Palpitations, sweating, anxiety, fear, chills, convulsions (hence contraindicated in status epilepticus), sweating, tachycardia
	• Re-sedation can occur due to short $t_{1/2}$ → Flumazenil doses may need to be repeated

Patient counselling	• *As drug is given in emergency situations or when the patient is sedated in the operating theatre, it is unlikely that patient counselling will be required; however, the prescriber should be aware of adverse effects, e.g. reversal of pain control, and be able to explain them if needed.*

Anti-Parkinsonian medications

Examples	• Co-beneldopa, co-careldopa, levodopa, ropinirole, pramipexole	
Mode of action	• Dopamine receptor agonists • Contain levodopa (precursor to dopamine) which helps to restore dopamine levels once converted to dopamine	→ In Parkinson's disease, there is a deficiency of dopamine
Routes of delivery	• PO, topical	
Indications	• Parkinson's disease (PD)	→ Can be initiated in early or late PD
Contraindications	• Contraindicated in breastfeeding • Caution in severe cardiovascular disease, convulsions, psychiatric illnesses, pregnancy and endocrine diseases, e.g. diabetes mellitus	→ Drug should be stopped in patients with exacerbated psychiatric conditions
Interactions	• MAOIs • Anti-hypertensive medications	→ Risk of hypertensive crisis → Potentiates hypertensive effect
Monitoring	• Discuss frequency of symptoms with patient • Monitor BP during treatment	→ To look for improvement in symptoms and quality of life → Due to postural hypotension

Side-effects	• Common:
	  – Nausea, vomiting, excessive daytime drowsiness, sudden onset sleep
	  – Dyskinesia
	  – Postural hypotension
	  – Psychological symptoms: dementia, depression, delusions, hallucinations
	• Rare:
	  – Levodopa is associated with impulse control disorders, e.g. gambling, binge eating and hypersexuality
		→ Majority of patients develop dyskinesia within 2 years of starting drug
		
		→ Increases risk of falls
		
		→ Levodopa should be withdrawn or reduced in dose until symptoms resolve

Patient counselling	• ***How to take:*** medication should be taken at the same time each day and patients or carers should be counselled on how to administer dispersible tablets, where relevant. • ***Do not stop taking drug abruptly:*** drug must be withdrawn gradually to prevent adverse effects. • ***Impairment of normal abilities:*** dopamine agonist drugs may affect ability to drive or operate machinery due to sedative effects. Excessive daytime drowsiness may occur. Do not drive or operate machinery if you feel dizzy or drowsy after taking this medication. Patients should be counselled on sleep hygiene. • ***Impulsive behaviour:*** warn patients on levodopa that it can cause problems with impulse control and the patient may find themselves doing things that are out of character. Advise patient to seek medical help, as drug needs to be withdrawn or stopped, and advise patient to seek social support. Safeguarding measures may also need to be implemented.	→ Abrupt withdrawal can precipitate dangerous conditions such as neuroleptic malignant syndrome or rhabdomyolysis.

Acetylcholinesterase inhibitors (AChEi)

Examples	• Donepezil, galantamine and rivastigmine	
Mode of action	• Prevent acetylcholinesterase from breaking down neurotransmitter acetylcholine • Donepezil is a reversible acetylcholinesterase inhibitor	→ Patients with dementia have a deficit of acetylcholine
Route of delivery	• PO, topical	
Indications	• Mild to moderate Alzheimer's disease	→ 1st line drug for this indication
Contraindications	• Use with caution in asthma and COPD, cardiac disease including sick sinus syndrome, susceptibility to ulcers and concomitant use of antipsychotic medication (increased risk of neuroleptic malignant syndrome) • Galantamine should be used with caution in GI obstruction	
Monitoring	• Drug should be reviewed at 6-monthly reviews	→ To decide whether to continue drug
Interactions	• Non-depolarizing muscle relaxants • Suxamethonium	→ Effects of AChEi may be opposed by drug → May potentiate effects of suxamethonium
Side-effects	• Side-effects tend to be dose-related so start at low dose and titrate up • Common or very common: – GI disturbances, e.g. nausea, vomiting, diarrhoea and anorexia – Muscle cramps – Headache – Dizziness – Rash – Pruritus – Syncope – Agitation – Hallucinations – Neuroleptic malignant syndrome	
Patient counselling	• **Explain effects of treatment:** • **General advice for keeping well:**	→ It is important to inform patient that drug will not reverse the pathological process that has occurred, maintain memory and function indefinitely or prolong the patient's life. → Provide general health advice that is useful for the dementia patient, e.g. eating a balanced diet, staying active, stimulating mind and socializing.

NMDA receptor antagonist

Examples	• Memantine	
Mode of action	• NMDA (*N*-methyl-D-aspartate) receptor antagonist, which increases the activity of neurotransmitter glutamate	→ Glutamate is involved with learning and memory
Routes of delivery	• PO	
Indications	• Moderate to severe Alzheimer's disease	
Contraindications	• Use with caution in severe hepatic impairment and in patients with history of epilepsy or convulsions or risk factors for epilepsy	
Interactions	• Levodopa, ropinirole, rotigotine, pramipexole • Ketamine	→ Memantine may increase effects of these drugs → Increased risk of CNS side-effects
Monitoring	• Mini-mental state examination (MMSE) should be repeated every 6 months • If score <10 and treatment with memantine deemed beneficial to patient, treatment should be continued	

Side-effects	• Common:
	  – Constipation
	  – Hypertension
	  – Dizziness and balance disorders
	  – Drowsiness
	• Less common:
	  – Heart failure
	  – Thrombosis
	  – Confusion
	  – Fatigue
	• Rare:
	  – Convulsions	

Patient counselling	• ***How to take drug:*** • ***Explain effects of treatment:*** • ***General advice for keeping well:***	→ Memantine should be taken at the same time each day. Patient should not stop taking drug on their own initiative. → It is important to inform patient that drug will not reverse the pathological process that has occurred, maintain memory and function indefinitely or prolong the patient's life. → Provide general health advice that is useful for the dementia patient, e.g. eating a balanced diet, staying active, stimulating mind and socializing.

Considerations when prescribing in the elderly:

- **Elderly patients make up the majority of hospital patients:** two-thirds of hospitalized patients are over the age of 65 and there is an ageing population as people tend to live longer. It is essential that prescribers should understand and adapt to the needs of the elderly population.
- **Physiological changes:** as an individual ages, their metabolism naturally slows down and many organs, e.g. the kidneys and liver, decline in function. This has an impact on pharmacodynamics and pharmacokinetics. Furthermore, elderly people are more sensitive to drugs that exert effects on the CNS (e.g. opioids) and may require lower doses than younger patients to achieve the same clinical effect.
- **Polypharmacy:** elderly patients are more likely to have multiple co-morbidities necessitating treatment with multiple drugs. The use of four or more drugs is known as polypharmacy. Polypharmacy increases the risk of adverse drug reactions, as the risk of drug interactions increases as the number of medications increases.
- **Risks associated with common drugs:** it is important to consider the impact of common drug side-effects such as constipation, dizziness and blurred vision on the elderly patient, who may already suffer from impaired functions. Anticoagulants are more dangerous in elderly patients than in young patients due to the increased risk of falls. Patients should receive full and comprehensive counselling regarding the risks and benefits of each medication they are prescribed, in order to make an informed choice about their treatment.
- **Antipsychotics in elderly patients:** the use of antipsychotics in the elderly has been linked with increased incidence of strokes, hence it is preferable to avoid prescribing antipsychotics to elderly patients.
- **Justify prescribing each drug and regularly reconcile medications:** it is important to have a clear rationale for why an elderly patient is being started on a particular drug, as they are more prone to adverse drug reactions and sometimes risk outweighs benefit. Performing regular medicines reconciliation helps to identify drugs that may be unnecessary.
- **Start low, go slow:** prescribe the lowest effective dose and slowly titrate dose up as tolerated.
- **Consider an appropriate formulation when prescribing:** some elderly people may have swallowing difficulties and those with severe rheumatoid arthritis may struggle to open the lid on some medication bottles. Work with pharmacist colleagues to optimize the ease of taking medications for the patient.
- **Memory and polypharmacy:** liaise with pharmacist colleagues regarding the use of blister packs to simplify self-administration of medications for elderly patients. Blister packs may be suitable for elderly patients who take multiple medications and may struggle to take their medications individually.
- **Prescribing in Parkinson's disease:** it is essential that medications to manage Parkinson's disease are not omitted or missed. Abrupt withdrawal of Parkinson's medications can cause life-threatening conditions such as neuroleptic malignant syndrome.

Section III:

Self-assessment questions and answers

Adverse Drug Reactions Item 1

ID ADR101

This question item is worth **2 marks**

You may use the BNF at any time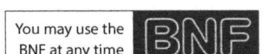

Case presentation
A 27-year-old woman with depression stopped taking her medication and developed a headache, shock-like sensations, paraesthesia and lethargy. She also complained of being unable to fall asleep.

Question
Select the ONE drug that is *most likely* to have caused her symptoms by being stopped. *(mark it with a tick)*

DRUG OPTIONS

A	Imipramine	☐
B	Olanzapine	☐
C	Paroxetine	☐
D	Sertraline	☐
E	Lithium	☐

Adverse Drug Reactions Item 2	**ID**	ADR102	This question item is worth **2 marks**	You may use the BNF at any time 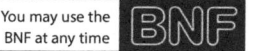

Case presentation

A 39-year-old man with diabetes and hypertension has recently been started on propranolol, in addition to his regular medications, to further reduce his blood pressure.

Question

Select the adverse effect that is *most likely* to be caused by this treatment.
(*mark it with a tick*)

ADVERSE EFFECT OPTIONS

A	He is at increased risk of hyperkalaemia	☐
B	He could develop palpitations at rest	☐
C	His glycaemic control may be impaired, making hyperglycaemia more common	☐
D	Signs of hypoglycaemia may be masked by propranolol	☐
E	He is at increased risk of bronchospasm	☐

| **Adverse Drug Reactions Item 3** | **ID** | ADR103 | This question item is worth **2 marks** | You may use the BNF at any time 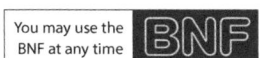 |

Case presentation

An 87-year-old man with schizophrenia and recurrent urinary tract infections has been admitted to hospital with pneumonia and is started on antibiotics. The following ECG is taken during his hospital admission.

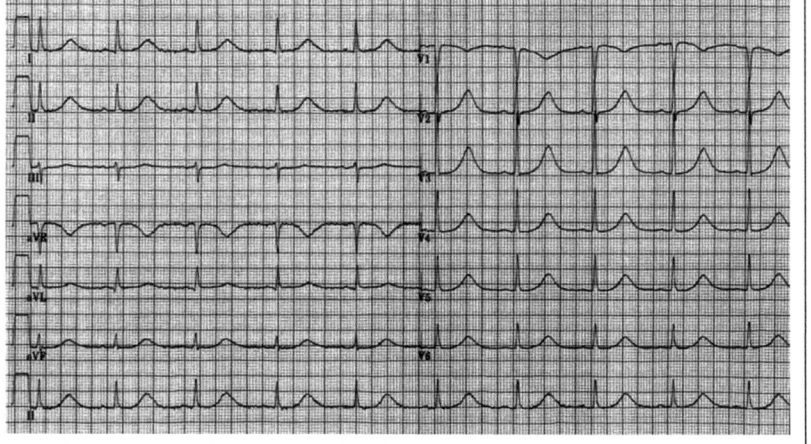

Reproduced with permission of Oxford Medical Education. Available at www.oxfordmedicaleducation.com/ecgs/ecg-examples/

Question

Select the ONE drug that is *most likely* to have caused the ECG appearance above.
(*mark it with a tick*)

DRUG OPTIONS

A	Amoxicillin	☐
B	Fluoxetine	☐
C	Clozapine	☐
D	Clarithromycin	☐
E	Nitrofurantoin	☐

| Management Planning Item 1 | **ID** | MAN001 | This question item is worth **2 marks** | You may use the BNF at any time 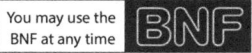 |

Case presentation

A 65-year-old man is brought to hospital by ambulance after developing right arm weakness and slurred speech. He was having dinner with his family at 6 pm when his daughter noticed that he struggled to lift his fork with his right arm and his speech was slurred. She became concerned when his symptoms did not resolve after an hour and called an ambulance. On arrival at the Emergency Department, the medical registrar examined the man and an urgent CT scan of the brain was requested. **PMH.** Hypertension. **DH.** Takes 5 mg amlodipine. No known drug allergies.

On examination

HR 105/min, BP 155/85 mmHg, SpO$_2$ 98% on room air, RR 14/min and temperature 36.3°C.

GCS 15/15.

The patient had marked right-sided weakness in his arm and leg and slurred speech; however, facial droop and visual field defects were absent.

Investigations

The CT scan of the brain showed no evidence of infarction or intracranial haemorrhage. This report was received at 11 pm and the patient's symptoms were still persistent.

Question

Select the *most appropriate* management option at this stage.

(mark them with a tick)

MANAGEMENT OPTIONS

A	75 mg aspirin	☐
B	75 mg clopidogrel	☐
C	40 mg enoxaparin	☐
D	4.5 mg fondaparinux	☐
E	300 mg aspirin	☐

Management Planning Item 2

ID MAN002

This question item is worth **2 marks**

You may use the BNF at any time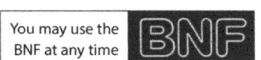

Case presentation

A 9-year-old girl is brought to the GP with a new rash. It was her sibling's birthday party the evening before; the girl developed the rash after eating birthday cake and she has been unable to stop itching. The rash has spread overnight. **PMH**. Asthma and atopic eczema. **DH**. Takes salbutamol and budesonide inhalers. Has peanut allergy.

On examination

HR 70/min, BP 115/75, RR 14, SpO_2 99% on room air and her temperature is 36.7°C. She is alert and playful, and is speaking in full sentences. On auscultation her chest is clear, normal heart sounds are heard with no murmurs present and her abdomen is soft and non-tender. She has a widespread blanching spotty rash over her trunk and legs.

Investigations

No further investigations were performed by the child's GP.

Question

Select the *most appropriate* management option at this stage.
(mark them with a tick)

MANAGEMENT OPTIONS

A	Prescribe chlorphenamine	☐
B	Give an IV injection of benzylpenicillin	☐
C	Give an IM injection of 1:1000 adrenaline	☐
D	Prescribe a steroid cream	☐
E	No intervention required (self-limiting problem)	☐

| **Management Planning Item 3** | **ID** | MAN003 | This question item is worth **2 marks** | You may use the BNF at any time | 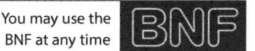 |

Case presentation
A 32-year-old woman presents with dysuria and increased frequency of micturition. She complains of mild generalized abdominal discomfort but denies nausea and vomiting. **PMH**. Otherwise well. **DH**. Takes the combined oral contraceptive pill.

On examination
HR 70/min, BP 115/75, RR 14, SpO$_2$ 99% on room air and her temperature is 37.0°C.

Investigations
Urinalysis shows +++leukocytes, ++nitrites but no blood or protein. The urine beta-HCG test is negative.
Her WCC is 11.2 and CRP is 12.

Question
Select the *most appropriate* management option at this stage.
(mark them with a tick)

	MANAGEMENT OPTIONS	
A	50 mg nitrofurantoin QDS	☐
B	200 mg trimethoprim BD	☐
C	625 mg co-amoxiclav TDS	☐
D	500 mg amoxicillin QDS	☐
E	Watch and wait approach	☐

Calculation Skills Item 1	**ID**	CAL001	This question item is worth **2 marks**	You may use a calculator at any time

Case presentation

A 5-year-old girl weighing 25 kg has fallen off her bike and she has fractured her right wrist. She is in moderate pain and requires regular 150 mg ibuprofen to be administered orally four times a day, in addition to the regular paracetamol she is receiving from her mother. The ibuprofen solution is available in 100 mg/ml.

Calculation

What volume of liquid should be administered for each ibuprofen dose?
(Write your answer in the box below)

Answer [   ] ml

| **Calculation Skills Item 2** | **ID** | CAL002 | This question item is worth **2 marks** | You may use a calculator at any time |

Case presentation

A 39-year-old man weighing 80 kg has attended the Emergency Department with a 3-day history of a painful and swollen right calf. He is otherwise fit and well and came back from holiday in Australia four days ago. A USS Doppler confirms a right leg DVT.

Calculation

What is the dose of enoxaparin that should be administered to this patient?

(Write your answer in the box below)

Answer [   ] mg

Calculation Skills Item 3	**ID** CAL003	This question item is worth **2 marks**	You may use a calculator at any time

Case presentation

A 13-month-old boy weighing 13 kg is brought to hospital following the development of a barking cough. He is seen by the on-call paediatrician who diagnoses him with severe croup and decides to prescribe a STAT dose of dexamethasone and observe the child for a response.

Calculation

What is the dexamethasone dose?

(Write your answer in the box below)

Answer [   ] mg

Prescribing Item 1

ID PWS101

This question item is worth **10 marks**

 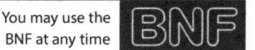

Case presentation
A 73-year-old gentleman has attended the Emergency Department with shortness of breath. He has taken his inhalers before attending hospital but is finding it hard to complete sentences. He denies chest pain and states that the shortness of breath came on when he was dusting his living room. He is apyrexial and has felt systemically well in the past months with no other symptoms. **PMH**. He is known to be asthmatic and has type 2 diabetes. **DH**. He takes metformin and has salbutamol and budesonide inhalers. Allergic to penicillin.

On examination
HR 110, BP 160/84, T 36.7°C.

Prescribing request
Write a prescription for a nebulizer that would be appropriate in this situation.
(Write your answer in the box opposite)

Answer

Prescribing Item 2

ID PWS102

This question item is worth **10 marks**

 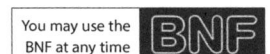

Case presentation

A 54-year-old gentleman with chest pain has been brought to the Emergency Department by ambulance. He describes severe central crushing chest pain, which started two hours ago and has spread to his jaw and his left arm. He has taken paracetamol and ibuprofen and he was given 2 puffs of GTN in the ambulance.

On examination

HR 110, BP 160/84, RR 20/min, SpO$_2$ 95% on room air and T 36.8°C. Pain score 8/10. Visibly distressed and clammy, clutching at chest.

Prescribing request

Write a prescription for a drug which may help to relieve the patient's chest pain.
(Write your answer in the box opposite)

Answer

Prescribing Item 3

ID PWS103

This question item is worth **10 marks**

 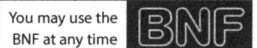

Case presentation

A 23-year-old man presents with angioedema and shortness of breath after accidental ingestion of peanuts at a restaurant. His partner noticed the angioedema and called the ambulance immediately. Unfortunately, the couple did not bring any of the man's medications with them to the restaurant.

On examination

He has angioedema to his face and throat. He is showing signs of respiratory distress but his airway is clear. There is no time to obtain a full set of observations as this is an emergency.

Prescribing request

Write a prescription for a drug that may help to relieve the patient's shortness of breath.
(Write your answer in the box opposite)

Answer

Extended Prescription Review	**ID**	REV001	This question item is worth **8 marks**

You may use the BNF at any time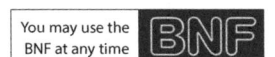

Case presentation

A 75-year-old woman with asthma, hypertension, type 2 diabetes and osteoarthritis has been brought to hospital following an asthma attack, which resolved following inhaler use. In the Emergency Department, bloods are taken and she is found to have a severe acute kidney injury which results in a hospital admission. She is noted to be mildly tachycardic, with a heart rate of 113, but her other observations are normal. She has been complaining of ankle swelling which she noticed over the past two months.

Question A
Identify the ONE prescription that is *most likely* to be the cause of her tachycardia.
(mark it with a tick in column A).

Question B
Identify the ONE prescription that is *most likely* to be the cause of her ankle swelling.
(mark it with a tick in column B).

Question C
Identify the TWO prescriptions that are *contraindicated* in view of her asthma.
(mark them with a tick in column C).

Question D
Identify the THREE prescriptions that are *associated with* renal impairment.
(mark them with a tick in column D).

CURRENT PRESCRIPTIONS

Drug name	Dose	Route	Freq.	A	B	C	D
salbutamol	2 puffs	INH	PRN	☐	☐	☐	☐
amlodipine	10 mg	PO	OD	☐	☐	☐	☐
ramipril	2.5 mg	PO	OD	☐	☐	☐	☐
aspirin	75 mg	PO	OD	☐	☐	☐	☐
metformin	500 mg	PO	BD	☐	☐	☐	☐
ibuprofen	200 mg	PO	BD	☐	☐	☐	☐

Adverse Drug Reactions Item 1. C. Paroxetine. Paroxetine is the SSRI with the shortest $t_{1/2}$, hence it is most commonly associated with serotonin discontinuation syndrome.

Adverse Drug Reactions Item 2. D. Signs of hypoglycaemia may be masked by propranolol. Beta blockers can reduce tremor and other signs of hypoglycaemia.

Adverse Drug Reactions Item 3. D. Clarithromycin. The ECG shows QT interval prolongation and clarithromycin is the most likely culprit.

Management Planning Item 1. E. 300 mg aspirin. The patient has suffered a stroke and there is no evidence of intracranial haemorrhage. The appropriate treatment is 300 mg aspirin as the patient is out of the thrombolysis window. It is advisable to give 300 mg aspirin PR, instead of PO, if the patient has not had a swallowing assessment performed and documented in the notes.

Management Planning Item 2. A. Prescribe chlorphenamine. The child has urticaria, a mild allergic reaction that results in a rash. Chlorphenamine will help to resolve the rash.

Management Planning Item 3. B. 200 mg trimethoprim BD. The patient has a confirmed UTI and she is not pregnant, so 200 mg trimethoprim BD for 2–3 days is an appropriate antibiotic course. Trimethoprim is the 1st line drug and if it does not work, nitrofurantoin can be tried.

Calculation Skills Item 1. 1.5 ml ibuprofen PO. This is a straightforward calculation.

Calculation Skills Item 2. 120 mg enoxaparin S/C. The treatment dose for DVT is 1.5 mg/kg and the patient weighs 80 kg; simple multiplication gives the dose 120 mg.

Calculation Skills Item 3. 1.95 mg dexamethasone PO STAT. For both mild and severe croup, the BNF advises 150 micrograms/kg for 1 dose. Dexamethasone is prescribed 150 micrograms/kg and if the child weighs 13 kg, simple multiplication gives the dose 1.95 mg (though not incorrect, 1950 micrograms STAT will not accepted as an answer).

Prescribing Item 1. 2.5–5 ml salbutamol NEB. Other acceptable answers include 2.5 ml or 5 ml salbutamol nebulizers.

Prescribing Item 2. 300 mg aspirin PO.

Prescribing Item 3. 0.5 mg of 1:1000 adrenaline IM. The other acceptable answer is 0.5 ml of 1:1000 adrenaline IM.

Extended Prescription Review. Question A. Salbutamol can cause tachycardia.

Extended Prescription Review. Question B. Amlodipine can cause ankle swelling.

Extended Prescription Review. Question C. Aspirin and ibuprofen can cause bronchospasm, so they are contraindicated in asthma.

Extended Prescription Review. Question D. Ramipril, metformin and ibuprofen can cause renal impairment.

With regard to patient safety, read the following statements and decide whether each statement is true or false.

1. A past medical history of migraines is a contraindication for the combined oral contraceptive pill.
2. When performing digital nerve blocks, it is safe to use lidocaine mixed with adrenaline.
3. Methotrexate should be prescribed through once-weekly dosing.
4. Treatment with levodopa is associated with impulse control disorders.
5. Levothyroxine should be taken 30 min to 1 hour before food or drink.
6. It is safe to administer 1 g paracetamol IV to a patient who weighs less than 50 kg.
7. NSAIDs should be avoided in asthmatic patients because bronchospasm can occur.
8. Factor Xa inhibitors can be reversed.
9. Tramadol causes more constipation and respiratory depression than codeine.
10. It is recommended that statins are discontinued 3 months before conception.
11. Nitrofurantoin causes a disulfiram-like reaction with alcohol.
12. Women who take oral contraceptive pills should use barrier methods to prevent pregnancy when taking antibiotics.
13. Splenectomy patients require long-term prophylactic antibiotics.
14. Trimethoprim should not be taken by pregnant women.
15. N-acetylcysteine can cause hypersensitivity-like reactions.
16. Lithium serum levels should be measured 8 hours after the last dose.
17. Tricyclic antidepressants, with the exception of lofepramine, are associated with the greatest risk in overdose.
18. Abrupt withdrawal of corticosteroids can cause an Addisonian crisis.
19. Activated charcoal is only indicated in patients who present to hospital within one hour of taking an overdose.
20. Adrenaline is administered via the IV route in anaphylaxis.
21. Patients who take amiodarone should take precautions to protect their skin from direct sunlight.
22. Adenosine is contraindicated in asthma and COPD.
23. Oral vancomycin is a potent antibiotic in systemic infections.
24. It is essential to aspirate before infiltrating with local anaesthetic to ensure that the needle is not in an artery.
25. Insulin should be administered subcutaneously, except in diabetic emergencies.
26. The efficacy of the combined oral contraceptive pill is not influenced by patient weight.
27. Patients with macrolide hypersensitivity can be be prescribed tacrolimus.
28. Fluoxetine is contraindicated in children.
29. The copper coil can be inserted as emergency contraception up to 2 days after unprotected intercourse.
30. In paracetamol overdose, serum paracetamol levels are measured 4 hours after ingestion (unless it was a staggered overdose).
31. Phenytoin is prescribed by weight.
32. Adenosine injection is a painful experience that patients should be warned about.
33. Enoxaparin is contraindicated in pregnancy.
34. Flumazenil is contraindicated in status epilepticus.
35. Oral vancomycin causes red man syndrome.
36. The use of antipsychotics in dementia patients has been correlated with a higher risk of stroke and death.
37. Sildenafil can cause sight loss.
38. Finasteride is not a teratogenic drug.
39. Calcium gluconate is prescribed in life-threatening hyperkalaemia.
40. In long-term NSAID use, a PPI should be taken to protect the gastric mucosa.
41. Naloxone administration can result in reversal of pain control.
42. The contraceptive implant is active for 2 years, after which it must be replaced.
43. Atropine doses may need to be repeated due to its short half-life.
44. Morphine is contraindicated in pregnancy.
45. Patients who are prescribed long-term steroids should be co-prescribed a PPI.

1. True. Women with migraines must not be prescribed the combined oral contraceptive pill.
2. False. Injection of adrenaline into organs with end-artery supply, such as the digits, is contraindicated.
3. True. It is a Never Event to prescribe methotrexate more frequently than once weekly.
4. True. This is an important side-effect to warn patients and their carers about.
5. True. Levothyroxine should be taken on an empty stomach, at least half an hour before food or drink.
6. False. A dose of 1 g of paracetamol in a patient who weighs less than 50 kg is a risk factor for paracetamol toxicity and this effect is more pronounced when administered via the IV route.
7. True. NSAIDs can, rarely, cause bronchospasm, which can be fatal in asthmatic patients.
8. False. At the time of writing, there is no reversal agent for Factor Xa inhibitors.
9. False. Codeine causes more constipation and respiratory depression than tramadol.
10. True. Statins can cause congenital anomalies.
11. False. Metronidazole causes a disulfiram-like reaction with alcohol.
12. False. According to the most recent guidance, barrier contraception should only be used if diarrhoea and vomiting occurs, which results in impaired absorption of the contraceptive pill.
13. True. Splenectomy patients must take long-term antibiotics as they are immunocompromised.
14. True. Trimethoprim is a folate antagonist.
15. True. In cases where hypersensitivity-like reactions occur, the BNF advises to reduce infusion rate or stop infusion until the reaction has resolved, and to treat symptoms.
16. False. Lithium levels should be measured 12 hours after the last dose.
17. True. This is one of the reasons why TCAs are not prescribed 1st line for depression.
18. True. It is important to counsel patients on this.
19. True. Although the use of activated charcoal has not been addressed in this book, it is important to be aware that it is only indicated in patients who present to the emergency department within 1 hour of poisoning.
20. False. Adrenaline should be administered via IM route in anaphylaxis.
21. True. Amiodarone can cause photosensitivity.
22. True. Adenosine can cause bronchospasm.
23. False. Vancomycin and teicoplanin are not well absorbed via the oral route so systemic infections should be treated via IV route.
24. True. This is crucial to ensure that adrenaline is not administered into blood vessels.
25. True. There are a few emergencies that indicate administering IV insulin.
26. False. Obese women may find that their contraceptive pill is less effective in preventing pregnancy, hence BMI over 40 is a contraindication for the combined oral contraceptive pill.
27. False. Tacrolimus belongs to the drug class macrolide although it is not an antibiotic.
28. False. Fluoxetine is indicated for treating depressive illness in children; however, this treatment would require close monitoring as the drug is associated with a small increase in risk of suicidal ideation.
29. False. The copper coil can be inserted up to 5 days after unprotected intercourse.
30. True. This is an important safety point, as serum paracetamol levels can be misinterpreted if measured earlier than 4 hours.
31. True. The patient's current weight must be known when prescribing phenytoin.
32. True. It is good practice to inform the patient that they might experience pain before the adenosine injection.
33. False. Warfarin is contraindicated in the 1st and 3rd trimesters of pregnancy, but enoxaparin can be used throughout pregnancy.
34. True. Flumazenil, rarely, causes convulsions, hence it is contraindicated in status epilepticus.
35. False. This is caused by IV vancomycin.
36. True. Antipsychotics should be avoided in those with dementia.
37. True. PDE5-inhibitors such as sildenafil can have adverse effects on vision.
38. False. Finasteride is teratogenic and precautions must be taken by individuals of both genders to prevent the risk of teratogenicity to an unborn child.
39. True. Calcium gluconate is administered in hyperkalaemia because it stabilizes the myocardium.
40. True. A PPI may reduce the risk of GI bleeding.
41. True. Naloxone reverses all effects of the opioid, including pain relief.
42. False. The contraceptive implant lasts for 3 years.
43. True. Atropine has a short half-life so bradycardia can recur and it is important to monitor the patient when administering atropine.
44. False. Whilst it is not recommended for pregnant women to take morphine, it is not contraindicated. However, pregnant women should not take morphine at term due to the risk of effects on the infant.
45. True. Similar to long-term NSAID use, long-term steroid use is associated with an increased risk of GI bleeding and thus, gastro-protection should be prescribed.

APPENDIX: MNEMONIC ACKNOWLEDGMENTS

Many people find mnemonics useful. Where existing mnemonics have been used in the book, the site where they can be found is given in the table below. Mnemonics listed with no source are the author's original work.

Mnemonic	Explanation	Source
ABCDE (antimuscarinic side-effects)	**A**norexia, **B**lurred vision, **C**onfusion/**C**onstipation, **D**ry mouth, **E**xpulsion of urine stopped (urinary retention)	
ABCDE (beta blocker CIs/cautions)	**A**sthma, **B**lock (heart block), **C**OPD, **D**iabetes mellitus, **E**lectrolytes (hyperkalaemia and metabolic acidosis)	www.medicalgeek.com/mnemonics/1482-pharmacology-mnemonics.html
ABCDEF	**A**rrhythmias/**A**nxiety, **B**lurred vision, **C**onfusion, **D**izziness/**D**iarrhoea, **E**mesis, **F**eeling nauseous	
ADP	**A**bnormal bleeding, **D**iarrhoea and other GI problems, **P**eptic and duodenal ulcers	
ASH	**A**ngina, **S**VT, **H**ypertension	
ASPIRIN	**A**sthma, **S**alicylism, **P**eptic ulcer/**P**remature closure of ductus arteriosus, **I**ntestinal blood loss, **R**eye's syndrome (in children), **I**ndigestion, **N**oise (tinnitus)	adapted from http://knowmedge.com/medical_mnemonics/Pharmacology_mnemonics/Aspirin:-Side-Effects/810
Can't see, can't pee, can't spit, can't shit		https://freepharmacyschool.com/2012/03/18/anticholinergic-memory-tricks/
CAPTOPRIL	**C**ough, **A**naphylaxis/**A**ngioedema, **P**alpitations, **T**aste disturbance, **O**rthostatic hypotension, **P**otassium elevated, **R**enal impairment, **I**mpotence, **L**eucocytosis	adapted from www.oxfordmedicaleducation.com/medical-mnemonics/pharmacology-mnemonics/
CHAT	**C**hurg–Strauss syndrome, **H**eadache, **H**ypersensitivity/**H**epatic disorders, **A**bdominal pain/**A**granulocytosis, **T**hirst	
CHEAP	**C**heese, **H**ydrolysed meats, **E**xtracts (yeast), **A**lcohol (wines, beers, low-alcohol drinks), **P**ickles, broad bean pods and banana skins	
COCP	**C**ycle control, **O**ccasional irregular bleeding, **C**lotting, **C**VD and **C**ancer (breast, cervical) more likely, **P**ain (breast tenderness, headaches)	
CODEINE	**CO**nstipation, **D**epression (respiratory), **E**mesis, **I**leus, **N**ausea, **E**xacerbates seizure activity	
COMA	**C**hronic alcohol abusers, **O**n drugs that induce cytochrome P450, **M**alnourished individuals, **A**norexic individuals	adapted from www.revise4finals.co.uk/medicine/mnemonics/r4f_pastest_mnemonics.pdf

CORTICOSTEROIDS	Cushing's syndrome, Osteoporosis, Retardation of growth, Thin skin – easy bruising, Immunosuppression, Cataracts and glaucoma, Oedema, Suppression of HPA axis, Truncal obesity, Emotional disturbances, Rise in BP, Oesophageal and peptic ulceration, Increased hair growth (hirsutism), Diabetes mellitus, Striae	adapted from www.oxfordmedicaleducation.com/medical-mnemonics/pharmacology-mnemonics/
CUSHINGOID	Cataracts, Ulcers, Striae and skin thinning, Hypertension, Immunosuppression, Necrosis (AVN of femoral head), Growth inhibited in children, Obesity/Osteoporosis, Increased hair growth (hirsutism), Diabetes	
DAMN	Diuretics, ACEi/ARBs, Metformin, NSAIDs	heard from a lecturer, but not published anywhere
DISCO	Digoxin, Isoniazid, Spironolactone, Cimetidine, Oestrogens	adapted from www.revise4finals.co.uk/cms/mnemonics/mnemonics/G
Don't Let you Fall a Sleep	Desloratadine, Loratadine, Fexofenadine, Cetirizine	https://forums.studentdoctor.net/threads/anyone-have-a-good-mnemonic-for-1st-and-2nd-gen-antihistamines.515892/
FAT MAP	Fine tremor, Anxiety, Tachycardia, Myocardial ischaemia, Arrhythmias, Palpitations/Pulmonary oedema	
GB	GI upset, Black tarry stools	
HMG CoA	Headache/Hepatotoxicity, Myalgia, GI disturbances, Complains of rust-coloured urine (rhabdomyolysis), Overproduction of serum liver enzymes, ALT rise (in particular)	adapted from www.medicalgeek.com/mnemonics/1482-pharmacology-mnemonics.html
IUCD	Infection/Incorrectly placed pregnancy (ectopic), Unintentional puncture (perforation), Crampy heavy period, Drop (expulsion)	
LITHIUM	Leucocytosis (rare), Insipidus (diabetes), Tremors, Hypothyroidism, Increased weight (weight gain), Urine excess, Mums beware (teratogenic)	
LMWH	Low platelets, More bleeding (haemorrhage), Weird reactions at injection site, Hyperkalaemia/Hypersensitivity/Hair loss	
METFORMIN	Metformin is a **big**uanide so you should give it to **big** people	
MORPHINE	Myosis, Out of it (sedation), Respiratory depression, Paralytic ileus, Hypotension, Infrequent opening of bowels and bladder, Nausea, Emesis	adapted from https://quizlet.com/36198507/pharm-mnemonics-flash-cards/
NALOXONE	Nausea, Agitation, LOss of pain control, eXcitation (restlessness), Opioid dependence, Neurological symptoms (fits), Elevated pulse rate	
NSAID	Nursing a baby (pregnancy and breastfeeding), Severe bleeding, Asthma, Issues with renal function, Drug allergy	adapted from http://dmnemonics.blogspot.co.uk/2012/11/contraindication-of-nsaid.html
PARK	Pregnancy, Allergy, Renal artery stenosis, K+ elevated (hyperkalaemia)	adapted from https://medmnemonics.wordpress.com/category/pharmacology/

PATCH	**P**ain (breast tenderness, headaches), **A**menorrhoea, **T**endency to put on weight (increased appetite), **C**lots and cancer more likely (breast, cervical), **H**ypertension (BP may rise)	
PCBRAS	**P**henytoin, **C**arbamazepine, **B**arbiturates, **R**ifampicin, **A**lcohol (chronic), **S**ulphonylureas	www.oxfordmedicaleducation.com/medical-mnemonics/pharmacology-mnemonics/
PHENYTOIN	**P**450 inhibition, **H**irsutism, **E**nlarged gums, **N**ystagmus, **Y**ellow-brown discoloration of skin, **T**eratogenicity, **O**steomalacia, **I**nterferes with folate metabolism, **N**europathy	www.valuemd.com/usmle-step-1-forum/13776-side-effects-phenytoin-mnemonic.html
POPs	**P**ain (breast tenderness, headaches), **O**veremotional (mood changes, premenstrual tension), **P**utting on weight (increased appetite), **S**potting or **S**top of periods (amenorrhoea)	
PPI	**P**ain (headaches, abdominal pain), **P**rone to catch C. diff. and get osteoporosis, **I**ntestinal (GI) upset	
Progestogenic IUS	**Progestogenic** (local) side-effects, **I**nfection/**I**ncorrectly placed pregnancy (ectopic), **U**nintentional puncture (perforation), **S**lipping out (expulsion)	
SSRIs	**S**ore tummy (GI upset), **S**exual dysfunction, **R**educed weight and reduced salivation (dry mouth), **I**ncreased risk of bleeding and convulsions, **S**erotonin toxicity and **S**erotonin discontinuation syndrome	
TCAs	**T**hrombocytopenia, **C**ardiac events (stroke, MI), **A**nticholinergic side-effects, **S**eizures	www.medicalgeek.com/mnemonics/1482-pharmacology-mnemonics.html
The 7 As	**A**ntibiotics, **A**nalgesics, **A**ntiplatelet drugs, **A**lcohol, **A**ntidepressants, **A**nti-pregnancy (oral contraceptive pills), **A**miodarone	
THYROID	**T**remor, **H**eart racing (palpitations), "**Y**ou may lose weight rapidly", **R**estlessness, **O**ut of character (mental/mood changes), **I**nsomnia, **D**iarrhoea	
VALPROATE	**V**omiting, **A**lopecia, **L**iver dysfunction, **P**ancreatitis, **R**etention of fat (weight gain), **O**edema, **A**norexia, **T**eratogenicity/**T**remor, **E**nzyme inhibition	www.oxfordmedicaleducation.com/medical-mnemonics/pharmacology-mnemonics/
Vomiting Patient Agreed To Have NG Tube	**V**omiting, **P**alpitations, **A**rrhythmias, **T**achycardia, **H**eadache, **N**ausea, **G**astric irritation, **T**oxicity	
Weight Gain Happens	**W**eight gain, **G**I upset, **H**ypoglycaemia	

INDEX

Bold indicates main entry